MW00943797

I Don't Care What You Eat . . . I'll Tell You What I Did!

I Don't Care What You Eat . . . I'll Tell You What I Did!

Daniel Alvarez

Copyright © 2013 by Daniel Alvarez.

ISBN:	Softcover	978-1-4836-9521-1
	Ebook	978-1-4836-9522-8

All rights reserved. No part of this book may be reproduced or transmitted in any form or by any means, electronic or mechanical, including photocopying, recording, or by any information storage and retrieval system, without permission in writing from the copyright owner.

This book was printed in the United States of America.

Rev. date: 10/14/2013

To order additional copies of this book, contact:
Xlibris LLC
1-888-795-4274
www.Xlibris.com
Orders@Xlibris.com
135948

CONTENTS

Introduction

My name is Daniel Alvarez, and I want to share the story of how I lost 320 pounds. There are 180 million people in the United States who are overweight, and my aim is to help as many people as I can. I have a crazy little dream that in the next hundred years or so, the number of overweight people in this country will become just 30 million, or even less. Someday, someone will say, "I read this book about this guy, two hundred years ago, who invented an amazing system that helped people to lose weight." I guarantee that whoever reads my book will be helped a lot.

I don't sell anything, nor do I want to teach anything. I just want to share my story. My point is that I once weighed 500 pounds.

Maybe you're a personal trainer, maybe you're a nutritionist, or maybe you're a doctor or psychologist, but you've never been 500 pounds. I respect the professionals so much, but I have the real experience of how I did it, and I want my experience to help others.

Always, helping people was a thing I had inside me, and I believe I've developed it for good. I never forget my degrees—I always say I have my master's degree in helping people and my PhD in loving people. For me, it's my life; that's why I'm living now. I promised God I would help people until the day I die, just like my idol, Roberto Clemente.

Roberto Clemente was one of the best baseball players in the history of baseball, and he was from Puerto Rico. He died going to help people. One of the worst earthquakes in Nicaraguan history was December 23, 1972. Five days later, Roberto Clemente decided to go help the people who had been impacted by the hurricane, and he died because he put too much medicine and clothes in the cargo hold of his airplane, which crashed. I would like to live, and die, just as my hero did, helping as many people as I can.

I think I was a born salesman. I remember that I was the most popular kid from an early age at school, and then in high school. I was the "class clown" guy. When Daniel moved, everybody moved. My concern all my life was to see people laughing, to see people smiling. What helped me in my high school have a lot of success also helped in my early days in sales. I sold encyclopedias at the age of fourteen years old (before there were computers) and I even sold light bulbs house-to-house when I was a Boy Scout. I thought that was a great business. Everybody needs light bulbs for their house, and when you take a lot of bulbs and go house-to-house, you can sell a lot of light bulbs for twenty-five cents apiece, even when you're eleven or twelve years old.

Every time I talk about my journey, I sell conviction. I guarantee 100 percent that when you get to the last page of my book, you will have learned from a lot of life. Maybe you're not going to lose the 300 pounds that I have, but maybe you're going to lose 10 pounds because that's what you need. My slogan is: I can help you from 1 pound to 300. Watch me. Of all the numbers between one and three hundred, I've lost that weight. A lot of people tell me they just want to lose five pounds, and I say, "That's simple. Let's go. Let's do it."

Helping people is a dream to me, and that is my goal for this book. When I see thousands of people reading the book and changing their lives, my dream will come true. I'm not an expert, I'm not a professional, but I can talk to people from experience. As I've said, my master's degree is in helping people, and my PhD is in loving people. Unless we can love people, this life will be different. God is amazing.

Sixty-five percent of people in the United States are overweight, and nine out of ten people fail at losing weight. Every single person has a focus, and you have to keep your focus forever. My focus is to change that number—I don't want to see nine out of ten people fail. Of the 65 percent of people that are overweight or obese, nine out of ten of them fail at losing weight for a reason, and I think the reason is either a lack of motivation or the fact that they don't know how to do it.

The diet and weight loss market advertises that people don't know how to lose weight themselves. The market convinces you that you have to go to professional people, and the professional people want your money and try to get the maximum amount of money that they can. If you fail, all they think is, *Oh, I'm sorry. Next!* I tell people they've got hope—for free—because no one can charge you to move. If you cannot walk or cannot swim, then you have to be careful what you're eating. If you cannot move, you're going to gain because you're not moving.

It's all in your mind. It's amazing how you can change your lifestyle in one second, but you have to want to do it; you have to believe in yourself. Not too many people are like me. Not too many have been 500 pounds and gone down to 185. There are a lot of shows about losing weight on TV, and a lot of people make money on all these shows. It's sad to say—and actually, I tell people not to do it—but try to find out where these people are after they win the prize, after the show is over. They go back again to being overweight. People who undergo surgeries to lose 100 pounds a day, or who select some other unsustainable method, they end up feeling miserable, or suffering.

Most people have to change naturally, and the natural way is to be consistent, persistent, and patient. Go slowly. Do the race of the turtle, not the race of the rabbit. The rabbit, I know, is going to fail. You're going to lose if you try to be a rabbit. But have patience, and everything you want is going to come. If you can envision something, you can accomplish it.

I used to be a big guy. I was just eating and eating and eating. My first two years working nights, I was eating during the day, eating at night, and then eating again at my home. I was never exercising, and that's why I was gaining my weight. You start gaining weight any time you eat a lot and don't exercise. Back in 2006 and 2007, I was 480 pounds. I believe I passed 500 pounds, but I didn't want to know it.

I'm an expert on weight loss now, and I discovered a lot of tricks. I call them tricks because in every seminar that I do, people want to know the tricks, the shortcuts. I always respect other people's professions, but I'm always honest with people, and I have to tell you, regarding psychologists, doctors, nutritionists, and personal trainers—anybody talking about charging people money to lose weight—I would make the same statement: if you have to pay money to lose weight, they're giving you advice because they want your money. I can prove that. I tried all the things that people try. I tried everything with no results. Obese people will tell me they are desperate to lose weight, and they will spend a lot of money because it seems like there's no other way. Inside, you always want to be healthy.

My daughter never did exercise for twenty-eight years, and she gained weight all the way to 397 pounds. Three pounds more, and she would have weighed 400 pounds. Today, she has been losing weight for almost one and a half years, and she's lost 160 pounds. I'm very proud of my daughter. She's doing a great, great, great job. The only change that she made was drinking more water and walking and swimming more (that is, getting in more exercise/physical activity). That's it. For a woman, losing 160 pounds is a lot. She's almost 240 pounds now, so she still has some work to do, but when you see the pictures, you see she's definitely made an amazing change.

Before she increased her level of physical activity, my sister also tried a lot of the same things that I've made allusions to earlier. Some of these weight loss techniques may have been effective at first, only to lose their effectiveness over time; others probably have never worked at all. Among the techniques: Weight Watchers pills, and the B12 shots, which are so famous here in Tampa, Florida. For a while, everybody was doing B12, and, working in the hotel, I knew a lot of housekeepers who did it. That was when I had lost 100 pounds already. "Danny, I invite you to do this B12," they said, but I told them to let me do it my way, which was natural. Now, all these girls are overweight again, and they lost all their money. I always love to be natural. Natural is walking; no one can charge you to walk. No one can charge you to drink water. Don't waste your money; you can do it yourself. I can tell you how.

Chapter 1

Find your "why"

If you want to lose weight, you have to find your "why." A lot of people who try to lose weight are doing it because someone told them to do it. *You're fat. You need to take care of your health.* It's all the people behind you, somehow urging you to lose weight. That doesn't mean anything. You need to know why *you* want to lose weight. Why do you want to do this? Is this going to be forever, or is this going to be for a movie or some party? Sometimes the reason is something like, *I need to lose twenty pounds for my wedding,* but that's not a real why, that's a temporary why. You need to know this is forever. *I don't want to be diseased; I want to look healthy for the rest of my life.* My why was my kids, my grandkids, and my health. That's what I figured out, and that's why I've been successful. I have not even gained two pounds back since I went from 500 pounds to 180 pounds.

You need to know your why. If you don't find the why, it's going to be tough. I don't want to say it's impossible, but it's close to impossible to lose significant amounts of weight if you don't know why you want to lose weight. Don't tell me it's because your friend told you or your neighbor told you or your husband or wife told you. It's you. The why is inside of you, and it's 95 percent related to families. Most of the people that I talk to have kids or grandkids, and that's the best type of why that you can have. Don't do it for them, do it for yourself, and they will be very, very proud of you.

The people on this planet of almost 7 billion don't even use 5 percent of their intelligence. God gave us all of our intelligence to use, but we use 5 percent of it, or less. The experts say that anyone who uses over 7 to 10 percent of their brain is a genius. These "geniuses" master life using just 10 percent of their intelligence—not 20, 30, or 50. Thus, if we want to do it, we can do it. My family said I use almost 10 percent of my brain. While I'm very humble, I'm also smart, and always use my logic. You must always learn first why you want to do something. If you don't find the why right away, my advice is to wait until you do, or you're going to lose time or money, and that could be worse for you.

If you make the decision to lose weight, you have to know how you're going to do it. Are you going to do it the easy way? Or are you going to do it the professional way? My professional way is forever. Just recently a woman told me she wanted to join a company that sells vitamins because they promised she'd lose twenty pounds in the first month.

"Congratulations. Try it, then come see me in twenty days," I said. A couple weeks later, I saw her again.

"Danny, you were right," she said. "I spent so much money, and I didn't even lose five pounds."

"Yep," I told her, "I know. These people just want your money, and I want your success. My success is your success."

In ten years, when you say, "I lost a lot of weight because Danny changed my life," that's my success.

Chapter 2

Puerto Rico and Florida: Starting a family

I was born in Puerto Rico on October 25, 1962. I was raised in a family of six people: my mom, my dad, two sisters, and one brother. I was raised in a nice family, a very Catholic family. We were always together, and I was raised like a normal kid. My mom was a housewife for almost fifty-three years, and my dad was always working in advertising agencies. Their anniversary is June 4. My parents gave me swimming lessons when I was four years old, and by the time I was five, I was swimming for fun. There are a lot of beaches in Puerto Rico, so we would spend time with the family on the beach and throw parties there almost every week. My parents were more concerned with me knowing how to swim than they were with any other ability of mine. My sisters and I studied in a Catholic school all the way through high school. My sisters were always involved in Girl Scouts and my brother and I were always in sports. It was the normal stuff that we do here in America. In 1973, when we were growing up, we were all together, always together. Now, after all these years, I have one sister living in Puerto Rico, and my other sister and my brother live here in Tampa.

I've always loved sports, and at the age of five years old, I was already swimming and playing baseball. I graduated from our swimming class before I hit kindergarten. Puerto Rico is an island, and there we love baseball, basketball, and any water sport, so I was raised in that atmosphere. At the age of nine years old, I started playing baseball, and I continued to do so until the age of seventeen. I've coached baseball for the past forty years, first in Puerto Rico and now in Tampa. I started coaching baseball in 1972, so it's been almost forty years helping kids in baseball.

As I've said, Roberto Clemente was my hero, my idol, and I remember very vividly how my life changed the day that he died. His legacy was everything to me because he helped kids in baseball, so I took from that legacy, and in 1972, I started coaching my brother. I was only eleven years old at the time, but I coached him until he was signed to a professional baseball team. I coached him at all levels from the time he was five to almost seventeen. In 1988, my son was born, and I coached my son almost until high school. So, I've always been involved with sports, and it's been part of my life to always help people.

I started my business, Daniel Printing, in 1984. I used to do any kind of printing, especially regarding posters and brochures. My main client was a travel agency that put out a lot of magazines. My printing company was very successful all the way through 1993 when I had to make my decision. In 1991, I was one of top industrial entrepreneurs in Puerto Rico at my age. I was twenty-six years old. I had my company in the best moment of my life, and it was a very successful company, but I stopped in 1993 to take care of my health.

I met my wife in 1988, and since that day we've been together. It's been twenty-five years now, and I still love her so much. She's been there through my good, my bad, and all the success I've had the last seven years. We're committed. Our daughter, Jennifer, was born in 1984. She's now twenty-nine. My son Daniel was born in 1988, so he's twenty-five years old now. Both of my kids have kids, so I have three grandkids. My daughter has two kids, and their names are Keith and Anthony. My son's son is a year and a half old, and his name is Kayden. He and I are always together. Every time we do something, it's always together. My kids are amazing, and for me, that powers my motor to do what I do.

My kids were very little when we decided to move, and we often visited the Tampa area. We'd go to Disney World, Busch Gardens, and all these places that kids love. It was as if I was almost psychologically preparing them for my decision, so when it was time to move, they were very happy. They didn't see any change at all, and I have no regrets regarding my kids having friends or their schooling in Florida. They've adapted since day one when we moved on June 1, 1995. Regarding the adaptation of my kids, I would use the term "extremely perfect." They're still here, so that means in eighteen years, they still love Tampa.

I was a super-healthy kid since the time I was born. All my years through high school, I was a sports guy. When I started my business, I gained a little bit of weight, but not too much. I'm six feet tall, so I was around 200 pounds, maybe 220. I was a normal person. But through my years of working so hard—ten, twelve, even fourteen hours per day—I used to get a little tired. I'll never forget that moment when I fell because I could not feel my legs. It was a little scary for me because I could not stand up, but I didn't pay too much attention to it. Then, a few weeks later, I felt the same symptoms and fell again. My hips went down, and I didn't feel it. That's when I made the decision to go to the doctor. It was the first time in many years. They discovered that I had muscular dystrophy in the first blood test. My muscles were getting weaker and weaker, and they had to do some treatment. Immediately, they did a biopsy for my muscles, but in less than three months, I knew that I was going downhill. The muscular dystrophy had already progressed so far. There are forty different types of muscular dystrophy. In 1952, Jerry Lewis started the muscular dystrophy telethon, which aimed to raise funds that could discover a cure for muscular dystrophy, but so far, we still don't have any cure. What was available at the time was treatment that could lengthen my life. In 1993, I started my treatment in Puerto Rico. I didn't feel any results, though, and I was feeling worse and worse.

Within two years, my health became very bad. I was almost in a wheelchair. I lost my company, and I had to make a difficult decision. One of my main doctors in Puerto Rico from the Muscular Dystrophy Association told me the best doctor then was not in Puerto Rico, but in Tampa, at the University of South Florida. So, I made the big decision to pack up my family, sell everything in Puerto Rico, and move to save my life. They predicted that I had four or five more years left to live; this was in 1993. That's when I made my decision with the help of my doctors.

My Doctor from Puerto Rico told me, "You have to make a big decision. You can continue your job, and you're going to die. Or you can choose to take care of yourself. You have little children, and I'm pretty sure you want your family."

In one second, I made the decision. I always tell people money is very important in life, but family is always first. It was almost twenty years ago, and I've never regretted my decision to save my life instead of continuing to make big business. In less than a year-and-a-half after they found muscular dystrophy in me, I was using a cane and then was confined to a wheelchair because I wasn't stable.

In 1994, I left Puerto Pico to come to Florida to continue my treatment. I've always been a positive person, so I told my family, "Let's go. Let's save Daddy's life," and we made the decision to move to Tampa in 1995. That's where my journey started with my health and my obesity.

The treatment here in Tampa saved my life. I was supposed to pass away in 1997, but being a positive person, I never paid attention to that. The only thing that I told the people in Tampa was just to save my life. I would do whatever I had to do. The treatment I received was a miracle, and the doctors cannot believe what I'm doing now. It was a big change for me to change my treatment, but I had confidence in the people at the University of South Florida in Tampa, especially my Doctors. She's been with me for the past ten years. It was a big change, but it was worth it because I'm still alive, and I'm getting stronger now. I'm doing everything better. The decisions I made were all worth it: I'm still here after 20 years.

In 1995, when I came from Puerto Rico, I was just taking care of myself. I was living to take care of my family with no job for almost five years. From 1995 all the way to 2000, I wasn't doing any work at all. I was just going to doctors and hospitals. Even though I was improving, at times, I had my downs. In five years, I stayed over ten times in hospital so that my blood clots could be dealt with, or I'd see improvements and then get weaker again. They were trying to get the best combination of treatments to keep me out of harm's way.

Around that time, I was getting a little heavier. One day in 2000, of the general managers of the hotel that I'm working at now offered to have me work for him part-time because he knew about my condition. I thought, *Well, let me talk to my doctors to see what they say. If it's something mentally that is going to change my life, I think it'll be okay.*

On June 1, 2000, I started working in a hotel in Tampa, and I've been there for the past thirteen years working part time as a driver. That's been another big change that happened in my life. So far, I'm still part time, but I'm happy with what I'm doing now. When we moved, I talked to my family. I said, "Daddy doesn't have a business anymore. We cannot have the same style that we're used to having in Puerto Rico." There, we had a pretty good standard of living. We had a great private school, a nice house, and everything. But my family adapted really well. They knew that Daddy was disabled and couldn't make much money. We survived with me working part time, my wife working, and public school. Like I said, money is very important, but it's not everything. Now, both of my children have families, and they live not even five minutes from me. They are always helping, and they support me. I don't see the money or the luxuries, but I am happy with my humble style. Looking back to my style back then, I would still say I'm happy with what I'm doing now.

Chapter 3

Obesity: Starting at the Hotel

I remember my first interview at the hotel. The human resources lady told me, "You have a job because the general manager says you have a job. Let me show you the hotel."

I'll never forget the first thing this lady showed me was the cafeteria for the employees. I exclaimed how nice it was, and she informed me the cafeteria is all-you-can-eat, free for all employees, all day and all night. *Wow*, I thought, *I've always loved to eat,* and I started eating and eating and eating, all day and all night. That's when I started to gain weight. In less than four years, between eating and doing no exercise, I went from 250 pounds to almost to 350 pounds.

Through my job, everybody knew me at the airport, and they were concerned about my weight because I was huge. One of the main grocery stores here in Florida is Publix, and Publix has a big weight scale that goes up to 300 pounds. For years, I would get on the scale and it would always say 300, even though my pants went from size 45 and 46 to 48 and 50. I was bigger than 300 pounds, but I thought in my mind I was 300 because that was as high as the scale went.

This guy in the airport told me, "We have a big scale here for luggage. If you want, you're welcome to try it."

I saw that I weighed 475 pounds, and that's when I got scared. I was super-heavy, and my waist was almost fifty-six inches at that time.

There were three important factors in my decision to lose my weight. The first one is my grandson. When he was two years old, he said, "Wow, Grandpa, you're so big."

The second one was my son's graduation. He asked me, "Daddy, can you wear a tuxedo in my graduation?"

I didn't find a tuxedo for almost two months. That's when I found out that I really was huge.

But, my main reason was a conversation I had with God. I was in my pool watching the sky, and I was talking to Him.

"God, what are you doing to me?" I asked Him. He was there, laughing. "Are you laughing at me?"

"Yes," He said, "I'm laughing at you. I saw you the other day looking on Google because you want to know how many people in this country are overweight. I can tell you the answer. There are 180 million overweight people here."

"Wow, that's almost 60 percent of the population."

"You're right, and you're one of the 60 percent. I know, Daniel, that your master's degree is in helping people. All the things we did together are coming down to you. My plan for you is that we're going bring that number down."

When I was searching the 180 million overweight people in this country, I also searched for the word *obesity* and found out about how many diseases you can have when you're obese. When I was big, my doctors could not believe they had a 500-pound person in front of them with no obesity-related diseases such as cholesterol, high blood pressure, or diabetes. Of all the diseases that people associate with obesity, I had zero, and I can prove it with the doctors' notes. I knew God was doing something to me, and I told Him that I knew and appreciated all He did for me. My condition had to do nothing with my obesity; my obesity was one thing and my condition was another. I was a huge person just preparing for my story.

I asked God, "What's your plan?"

"Danny, don't worry," He said. "I know you love people, and I know you want to help people. We are going to do something together, but I want you to promise me something."

"Anything you want me to promise, I'm going to say yes."

"I want you to start helping people with your story," He said.

"That's a good deal. I love to help people." I asked Him how.

"Look down," He said, and I looked at my body in the pool. "That's where we're going to start. Swimming."

Water is something that people don't have any idea what it means outside or inside their bodies. I remember swimming at my own house, just on my patio. I am lucky to have a big swimming pool. I started swimming and swimming, all day and all night. I remember my joints and my muscles were getting stronger, and I was feeling much better. At the same time, I was losing weight.

I remember the first year when I lost my first 50 pounds. It was 2007 or 2008, and I weighed 450 pounds. It was during the Olympics, and I'll never forget Michael Phelps in an interview on ESPN. He was telling people that he eats ten thousand calories a day, but to win all these gold medals, he had to swim four or five hours a day. I thought, *Hold it. That's me. I love to eat, and I love to swim.*

When people ask me what was my change in food, that's when I tell them one of my tricks. If you talk to a nutritionist, the first they're going to start cutting is certain foods. I respect the professionals, but I'll tell you something: when you take food out of the system of an obese person, nine out of ten people are going to fail. I tell people not to concentrate on the food and to concentrate on the exercise.

God told me, "Remember, people forget that I created people to be able to burn calories."

I discovered this at a moment when I had lost over 200 pounds and hadn't changed my diet at all. The only difference that I made in my life was that I started doing some exercise. I've discovered that the more exercise you do, the more you can eat. That's how human beings work. Ninety-five percent of the people I talk with are obese, and they can connect with me because I've been there. Psychologists say that 20 to 31 days in a row makes a habit, but in my book, that is not true. To make weight loss a habit, you need 365 days. You don't have something that's a positive habit until you have been doing the same thing at about the same level of intensity for about 4 or 5 months.

There are a lot of people in the gym at the YMCA I go to on January 1, but by February or March, they fail. There's a lack of motivation to do something, and it's understandable because it's hard to change your lifestyle, but that's the most successful thing that I did. I changed my lifestyle from day one. I changed from one thing to another thing, but I never touched the food. The food is something you have to learn through the process. The more you start losing, the more you can eat whatever you want. I don't care what you eat; you just have to tell me how much exercise you do. As soon as you tell me how exercise you do, then I can tell you why you are overweight.

I try to concentrate on people with obesity, which is a lot of people. Over five hundred people have had success with my system, which is to concentrate first on the exercise. They ask, "Daniel, can I eat anything I want?" *Yes!* When people call food trash food, garbage food, junk food, I have to tell them straight: I'm mad when I hear that. Food, for me, is sacred. We're talking about 2 billion people in this world who don't have food, so don't call food "junk food," "trash food," or "garbage food."

For me, it's healthy food or lesshealthy food. That's all you can tell me about food. You can choose to eat healthy foods or less healthy foods. Ultimately, you have to do more exercise if happen to love less healthy food and eat more of that. If you eat more healthy food, you may not have to do as much exercise.

Chapter 4

Weight and exercise: Types of People

There are four kinds of people on this planet when it comes to weight and exercise. I don't care if they're celebrities or if they're homeless. There are the ones who eat healthy and exercise, the people that eat healthy but don't exercise, people who don't exercise and don't eat right, and then the last group that loves eating and doing extreme exercise. Sometimes, they might do too much exercise and won't eat too well; other times, they eat healthy but don't exercise. You have to know which kind of person you are. The healthiest people are the ones in the first column, who both eat healthy foods and also exercise.

I explain to people that we come like a package. When you're born—and this is going to blow your mind—you gain one pound every single month until you turn one year old. I always wondered why that is. I know babies eat super-healthy. The mother's milk is very nutritious, as are all the formulas that Gerber and all these companies make, but babies will gain because all they do is sleep and eat. Eat and sleep. Sleep and eat. They do this all day and all night for nine, ten, eleven, up to twelve months. And what happens in a year? After a year, they're probably crawling, maybe walking, and we call that exercise. It's not a coincidence that even babies eating healthy will gain pounds for not moving. When babies stop eating nutritious milk or formulas, they get super-active so they don't gain more. They might be eating less healthy foods, but they're so active, they don't gain.

Fat comes when you don't move. I have my theory that if you don't want to exercise, then you have to eat healthy, but if you don't want to eat healthy, you have to move. Even if you're eating healthy, you still have to move to burn calories. Thank God we can burn calories. You burn calories every day, even sleeping. Babies don't do anything at all, just sleep and eat, but what would happen if we weren't able to burn calories? In my case, in a day, I can eat two thousand calories. In a month, that means I can eat sixty thousand calories. How much is sixty thousand calories? It's over fifteen pounds. By fifty years old, then, I should weigh over 1,600 pounds. If we couldn't burn calories, we'd keep gaining and gaining, even if we eat healthy like babies do. Healthy food also has calories, and it seems like a lot of people don't know that. So, if you've been eating and eating without burning calories, then by the age of fifty, you would weigh more than 1,500 pounds. That's a lot.

Of course, I'm not 1,500 pounds, and that's because after one year of age, you start moving and burning. Some people burn more, some people burn less, and some people don't burn much, but every person is capable of burning calories. Babies have fat because they don't move. They call it "baby fat" because the little body is just receiving calories, even healthy calories, without doing exercise. You're never going to see a one-month-old or a two-month-old walking, because it's a process, and process, for me, means at least one year to make a habit.

The nutrition people say, "Yeah, that's good logic. That's why babies are babies."

Can you imagine at one day old if a baby starts getting unhealthy food? They're going to gain more than normal. As soon as babies can walk, they start eating more unhealthy stuff, but they gain no more than ounces in a month because they're moving. They gain because they're getting taller, but the fat of babies and the fat of adults is almost the same depending on how active they are during the day, and what kinds of activities they do.

Everything starts at the beginning of your life and depends on how you treat those first 5 years. I can show you a picture of me holding my swimming diploma at five years old, a super-skinny kid. Whoever said that if you're born fat, you're going to be fat all your life? That's not true. When I was born, I weighed almost eleven pounds. My mom always had a joke that after two weeks, she couldn't hold me because I was so huge. After that, by the age of five years old, I was a very skinny kid. But that's because I was swimming when I was three, four, and five years old.

For these reasons (the fact that whether I was skinny or fat had so much to do with activity), I'd say that when people concentrate just on the food element of weight loss, they fail to lose weight. That's why 90 percent of Americans can't lose weight: it's all based on food. Pills, diets, advertising on television, products. But they don't exercise. If you're 30, 50, or 80 years old, unhealthy eating and the absence of exercise leads to weight gain. Let's then focus on the kinds of food and the amount of exercise, and not strictly on the amount of food. Let's accept that, as we get older, we may need to change our habits to keep weight off.

Regarding food, I add, rather than eliminate, more stuff in my diet. Puerto Rican people, Latinos, we have our rice and beans and pork chops, and I never eliminated those. I love sandwiches, and I'm addicted to sandwiches, and I eat anything I want. But as soon as I eat it, I burn it. I never forget when God told me, "Daniel, don't forget how I made you." You don't have to suffer eating. That's the major reason people fail because they change their habit of eating. They do diets, and I don't trust in diets.

"Danny, can I do this diet?" people ask.

"Are you going to do it for the rest of your life?" I say.

If the answer is yes, I say do it, but if they say no because they told me it's just a thirty-day diet or a one-week diet to lose 10 pounds or whatever, I say, "Yeah, but what happens when you stop? You're going to gain it back."

The lifestyle that people start as soon as they start my system is forever; you can never stop it. We learn through the process. I've learned that the better I eat, the less exercise I have to do. When you're born, you come with a package. In my case, at six feet tall and fifty years old, the calories that God gave me for free are 1,700 calories, up to 2,000, in one day. That package means that if I don't eat more than 1,700 calories, I'm not going to gain. If I eat less than 1,700 calories, I'm going to lose weight, so between 1,700 and 2,000 calories, I'll be stable. I know a lot of people who always stay in the same pattern for years because they eat the same package. So why do people gain? I gained because I was eating around 3,000 calories, and of course, my package never changed. I'm always going to be six feet tall. My grandkids change every year because they grow taller and taller, but adults stop growing. My package of calories is still the same. I gained because my average was 3,000 to 4,000 calories in a day, and that's almost double what my package allows. When you eat a total of 3,500 calories more per week above what your package is (for example, if your package was 2,000 calories a day, but you ate 2,500 a day, you'd eat 3,500 extra calories), that would lead to gaining one pound.

Everybody has a package, and the key to managing your package is exercise. So far, no one has been able to tell me any one food from around the world that will kill you if you eat it. We're talking about food, not poison. Healthy, unhealthy, whatever you call it, you cannot eat food and die immediately unless you have an allergic reaction. You die with unhealthy food if you, like I did, for almost seven years, eat unhealthy food and do zero exercise. That's how you gain weight. I will gain weight whether I'm eating Italian food, Latino food, American food, or eating healthy if I'm not exercising. On the flip side, I can still lose weight eating healthy foods, vegetarian food, Latino food, or American food. Food is not the problem. The problem is when you eat it and leave it in your system for more than twenty-four hours. It's a problem when all the salts, fats, and sugars build up. It's important to avoid leaving food in your system for more than twenty-four hours.

Food is not the problem, and that's why I say not to concentrate on the food but just to concentrate on the exercise. When I tell people to eat anything they want, they love me. I don't touch the food; I just touch the exercise. I lost my first 200 pounds by swimming and not changing my food. When I got to 300 pounds, I got a little stuck. I was stuck for almost three months, just passing the 300-pound mark. I thought, *wow, what happened?* And that's another thing that I try to explain to people. You have to have a plateau. It's impossible that you won't have this plateau, and you have to figure out what you have to do. I already swam all day, so I started walking. In my article in the Huffington Post, the title says, "Daniel Alvarez Lost 280 Pounds by Walking and Swimming." That's real. I started just by swimming and walking. When I started walking, I'd walk for maybe one mile. After a while, I thought, *That's not enough,* so I'd go two miles, and then I'd switch to swimming. I can say that through swimming and walking, I lost 300 pounds.

You can check out my video on Google, just search for "DANIEL ALVAREZ FOX 13" and "weight lost."

Chapter 5

The scale

The professionals might tell you otherwise, but I say it's important to have a scale. The trainers tell you not to go to the scale because you get crazy, but I find that most people don't know how much they weigh. One hundred percent of the people maybe think they know how much they weigh, but when we go to the scale, I prove almost every day at the YMCA that they don't. Your second or third friend in the journey to weight loss is the scale. You need to know daily—or twice a day, even three times a day—how much you weigh. As soon as you know in the morning how much you weigh, in the afternoon how much you weigh, and at night, you're never going to gain more than two pounds because you'll be in control of yourself.

They will tell you to weigh yourself once a week, but you can easily gain five pounds in that one week. To get back five pounds, you have to lose 18,000 to 20,000 calories, and that's a lot. People don't know how much they weigh, but if I ask how much gas is in their car, every single person knows the answer. How can you know your car but not know yourself? Obviously, we don't have a gauge or a meter to know how much we weigh like the car, but that's why we have to use the scale every day.

Say we fill up your gas tank, and I take the front panel of your car out so you don't know how much gas you have. How do you think you're going to drive after the second day, the third day, or the fourth day? That's the same way that you do yourself. If you don't know how much gas you have in your tank, that's when you get crazy. It's the same thing with your body. You need to know how much you weigh on a daily basis. Nine out of ten people who don't use the scale will gain, but the people who use the scale every day will have success with my system.

You cannot weigh the same amount all day. Normally, obese people can gain two or three pounds in one day, and also lose two or three pounds in one day. My best motivation, as I tell people, is the scale. Let's say I'm 185, and when I get on the scale and am 184, believe me, I'm going to be very happy. But if I'm 187 or 188, my brain is going to say, *Oh, let me control myself. Let me walk a little bit more, let me swim a little bit more. Let me exercise a little more.* You control yourself on a daily basis. A lot of people at the YMCA exercise Monday through Friday, and then Saturday and Sundays they take off. Then, they come back again on Monday, and they've gained one or two pounds because they didn't do anything Saturday or Sunday.

The other important tool in weight loss is drinking water. From day one when I was born all the way to my forty-fourth year, the gallons of water I drank would probably not even come close to the amount of water I've been drinking for the past four or five years. Drinking water is an absolute miracle for weight loss, and it's the most major change I made in my diet.

Sometimes you don't have quite enough time to exercise, but I know a trick. Sometimes you need money, so you go to the bank, and the bank lends you money. When you don't have time to exercise, borrow some time from your sleeping time. I don't care how much you sleep, just borrow one hour. We have 1,440 minutes in a day. Out of that 1,440 minutes, take 40 for you. Don't tell me that you don't have time. Maybe you don't have the commitment, maybe you don't have the dream, maybe you don't have the support, but you have the same amount of time that everyone else does.

There are a lot of reasons that people fail. This society has complicated life so much. Everything is about rushing, about money. There's no more value of families, no more eating dinner together. We have to see this life simply. It's just life. Every single person on this planet is a baby. When eighty-year-olds tell me they're too old for something, I say, "Hold it. Eighty years old? We're in 2013. Divide eighty years by 2013 and see your results. It's 0.04. That's how long you've been living on this planet. It's nothing. You're a baby." To tell me that you're too old to do something for your health, you have to at least convince me that you're 2,000 years old. If we're in 2015, and you're 2,000 years old, then maybe you're old. But even then, the sun is 4 billion years old and is still bright. You have to look at this life in another way.

When anyone asks me how I'm doing, I have just one answer. No one can catch me with another answer. I say, "I'm always good." *How you doing, Danny?* "I'm always good." Especially at five o'clock in the morning, driving airline crew members to the airport. "How you doing, Danny?" they ask. "I'm always good." I have to enjoy my life. It's just one that you get, and you don't know when you're going to die, right? I tell people sometimes to think about the second they know they're going to die. If you know the date that you're going to die, you're going to change your life immediately. I don't care if it's in the next five years or the next twenty years, but as soon as you know that you have the finish line, you're going to change your life.

Why don't we think like that every day? I'm talking to you today, but I might not be talking to you tomorrow. If I die today, I'll be very happy with all the hundreds of people I've helped already. This journey is going to be expressed around the world because I've had that hope. I know that I'm going to touch a lot of people with my system because it's almost 90 percent mind. We are overweight because something happened in our minds. There's some problem, some stress, whatever. We have to work in our mind by starting with the logic stuff. Be smart and use your brain, not your head. The brain is so capable, and we don't even know how far it can go. The brain automatically comes with your habits that you've had all your life.

For example, say there's two salesmen, and one is very positive while the other is very negative. I discover an island with 1 million people, and those million people are barefoot. No one has shoes, and my two salesmen sell shoes.

One salesman says, "I'm going to be a millionaire! I'm going to sell at least a million shoes over there!"

The other one says, "You know what? No one has shoes. They don't want to buy shoes."

The brain of the positive person thinks differently than the brain of the negative person in the same situation considering the same people, the same island, and the same shoes. Why is that? It's because the positive person can see a lot differently than the other person with the same situation. Ask yourself why you want to lose weight and envision yourself 20, 30, or 40 pounds less. Put it in your brain. Remember about the geniuses that use 10 percent of their brain? We're capable of going past the 10 percent, but some people just don't believe they can. Some types of people don't see it.

One example I give people is this: Close your eyes. Right now, we're on the beach with our family. Nice breeze, sunny day. It's one of the most beautiful days. Your piña colada is right there. You see your kids playing on the beach. Now, see the sky in your brain. What do you see in the sky? You see an elephant, and that elephant is pink, and it's coming toward you.

The elephant is yelling to you, "Hi! Hi Diane! How are you doing?" You cannot believe what you are seeing.

"Watch that elephant! It's coming to us!" you tell your kids. The flying elephant comes down, lands on the beach, and starts talking to you.

"How are you? Are you having fun?" says the elephant.

"Yes," you say, "but how can you fly, elephant? How can you talk?"

He says, "You know what? You're going to find out later," and the elephant starts flying back through the sky, and you see him very far away.

Now, open your eyes. What person didn't see the elephant? What person didn't see the scenario? Pretty much everyone always says that they saw it. Last time I checked, seeing a flying elephant is impossible.

See how far your brain can go? Your brain is able to go beyond whatever the first or typical think you think of is.

People have to use their brains to get anything they want in this life. I always challenge a person to give me a dream that no one has on this planet. If it's a dream and you have it, it's because you saw it or you want it because someone has it. Dreams come true in your brain, and they move from your brain to your heart. If you live in your brain, and keep the dream locked there, the dream will simply stay in your brain and not manifest in the real world. But if you move the dream from your brain to your heart, it will become something you can attain. The billionaires in the United States are billionaires because they had a dream, and they started working for that dream. The majority of people don't make their dreams come true because they don't put it in their hearts. The brain is different than the head. Your head is your head, but you have to use your brain for anything that you want. If you want to lose weight, you use your brain and your logic.

I say your brain can go so far that you see an elephant fly. Ask yourself, what's your dream car? What's the car that you want but don't have? People usually respond to me with a lot of cars: Bentley, Lamborghini, whatever. Do you think if we go to Italy and see the Lamborghini Company, do you think we're going to see one Lamborghini per second built in there? Do you think the Lamborghini Company is stupid enough to make a Lamborghini with no reason? Someone's going to have a dream, and they're going to realize it. Any dream that you have—any dream—you can have.

The difference between the people who make dreams and the people who don't make dreams is that transfer from brain to heart that sometimes takes an entire lifetime. When Bill Gates dreamed of leaving Harvard to found Microsoft, he had that dream, and he started doing that. Dreams come true as soon as you put them into work. The brain is amazing. If I say, "Don't think of a horse right now," you'll still be thinking of a horse right now. The reason why is because the brain goes straight to that thought. It's part of being smart. Use the brain, not the head.

Chapter 6

CPP: Consistent, Persistent, and Patient

CPP is my most important motto. I invented CPP in my head, which stands for consistent, persistent, and patient. If you pick one of the three and take it out of your system, I'm sorry, but it's going to be hard to lose weight that way. You have to embody *all three* of the words that go into CPP. The biggest reason that people who try to lose weight fail and get frustrated is because they don't have patience. My strategy for getting down from 500 pounds was not rushing, not having any date that I wanted to reach my 185. I was able to be extremely patient. It's the race of the tortoise and the hare again. Be patient, and you will win the race. Let the rabbit go as far as it wants, and you just go as fast as you can. As soon as you do this, your patience will get stronger and stronger.

Unless you set goals, your patience will only grow more. That's why I tell people not to set goals. Don't tell me that you want to lose twenty pounds in three months. Tell me that you want to lose five pounds in three months, and it will come, as soon as I explain to you how I do it. You must put pressure on yourself to have the patience that you must have, and to have the consistency and persistence that goes along with it. You can have persistence, but if you don't have patience, you're going to fail.

Patience and persistence without consistency is evident in the people who say, "Oh, I'm going to exercise twice a week or three times a week." That doesn't work; it has to be every day. You're capable of sleeping every day. You're capable of eating every day. You're capable of going to the bathroom every day. Why wouldn't you be capable of exercising every day? It scares me that professional people tell everyone not to exercise every day. You don't have to do extreme exercise every day—it all depends on how much you eat the day before. Today, I did just one hour of walking. That's normal, and that's okay—I did something.

When I give my talks, I hold up four fingers to make my point. With the first finger, I say, "Do you eat every day?"

Everybody says, "Yes, I eat every day."

"Perfect," I say. "Do you sleep every day?"

"Oh yes, I sleep every day."

"Okay, that's perfect. Do you go to the bathroom every day?" That's the third finger.

"Yes, I go to the bathroom every day."

Then I say, "You don't exercise every day, right?"

"No," they answer, "I don't exercise every day."

"Let me rephrase this question then. What happens if I tell you—and try to convince me—not to sleep for the next ten days?"

"That's impossible."

"No problem, but then don't eat for the next thirty days."

"Danny, that's impossible."

"I agree. How about you try to not go to the bathroom for the next year? See what happens then."

"Danny, that's impossible!"

"So that's impossible. But if I tell you don't exercise for ten years, you say, 'Oh yeah, I can do that.' Oh really, so that's an option?"

For the first three fingers, they come along with your life. No one has to tell you that you have to sleep, or you have to eat, or you have to go to the bathroom. That comes in your life. Why is the fourth finger—exercise—an option? Why do you choose yes or no? I tell people not sleep for three days, and they say that's impossible. So why not put this fourth finger together with the other three?

People ask me, "Danny, you exercise every day?"

"Yes," I tell them. "Just like I eat every day, like I sleep every day, like I go to the bathroom every day."

I don't do the same exercise every day, just like you don't eat the same thing or the same amount every day. You don't sleep the same exact number of minutes and seconds of every day—sometimes you sleep more, sometimes you sleep less, right? You don't go to the bathroom exactly three times or forty times. It's always different, and exercise is different. Don't cut the exercise part of your life. If you don't like that part of your life, then we have to talk about eating. You have to eat healthy, and you can't surpass your package. As long as you don't surpass your package, you're never going to gain. You only gain because you surpass your package.

The CPP is very, very important. You have to be consistent. No one tells you when you have to sleep; it's automatic. When you lose the weight, you still have to be persistent, and you must be patient. This is forever. Patience is something that you must have in your mind. Success doesn't come easily, and it's easy come, easy go. In my case, I believe seven years is enough.

A lot of people tell me, "Danny, I have to lose 10 pounds this week."

"Don't worry," I say. "Have another week."

"Oh Danny, I didn't lose one pound the entire month," they complain

"Okay, so take another month," I say. I have a lot of patience.

People laugh, but I like to tell them that 2014 is coming and 2016 is coming. 2050 and 2100 is coming, though none of us may be around to see either of these years. You cannot concentrate on the dates. The date that you finish is the date that you die.

You have to have CPP all the time. In Spanish, it's also CPP: *consistencia, pasciencia, persistencia.* That means that you're positive, and you're consistent. You're doing at least something every single day. I know you're capable of going one day without eating, or that you can stay up for twenty-four hours. You don't want to die, though, so you don't do these things voluntarily all the time. I don't know if can go one day without going to the bathroom. But exercise, that's what people choose. Say you eat for two or three days and don't exercise. In those three days, you just eat, and what happens? You're going to pass your calories package, guaranteed 100 percent. If you eat three days, you're going to pass your 3,500 calories that make a pound. Even eating 1,900 calories a day, without exercise you'll gain about a half pound in three days. Even eating a little bit, if you don't burn while you eat, you're going to gain. That's what I know. It's scary, but 180 million people in this country are like that. They don't concentrate on what they have to do, on burning what they have in their system.

The hardest part of CPP for people is the last word, *patience.* Pretty much everyone who makes a decision to lose weight is motivated on that day they make their decision. But for how long will they be motivated? Are they the match, the candle, or the torch? Maybe they're going to do it the first week, but like I said, to be consistent, you have to do something for at least six months. Consistency is when I see people walking with me, walking the trail, or going to the YMCA for six months in a row without missing more than one day or maybe missing the weekend. If I see them Monday through Friday, that's consistency.

Persistence is when you keep trying. I ask people how many pounds they've gained in the past 10 years. They tell me they gained 20, 30, or even 40 pounds. If it took that long to gain the weight, you're not going to lose those 30 or 40 pounds in one day or two weeks. It can take a year, five years, ten years—be fair to yourself with your gain. Put three or four years back, and don't try to lose all the weight because you're desperate. Be persistent, and you will see results.

Have patience. Patience is the most important thing people have to have if they want to lose weight. If you don't have patience, if you're frustrated because you fail to lose weight at a satisfactory pace, I guarantee it's because you set goals for yourself that you couldn't meet. Goals are your enemies. Goals are for sports, but dreams are for you. Dreams are different than goals. If you say you have a dream to lose 20 pounds, I'll back you up.

The last time I lost patience with myself was the day before I decided to lose weight. I've had complete patience since the moment I made the decision to lose weight when God told me we were going down together. My frustration comes when I see people who are motivated for one day but their candles go out the first week. Habits come after a year. It took a long time to form the habits you already have, so it's not twenty-one or thirty days (like many psychologists seem to think). To lose weight, you need a year, and you must be both consistent and persistent in order to do it. I get frustrated with people who aren't motivated enough.

Another pillar of my system I call the QQ. The QQ stands for *quality* versus *quantity*. You choose the quality of food you're going to eat based on the quantity of exercise you want to do. One is based on the other. If you have the same amount of quality of food and the same amount of quantity of exercise, you're going to break even. That's good, and when people come to me and tell my they didn't lose even one pound, I tell them that's awesome because maintaining your weight is also a success. Sometimes they'll tell me they lost one pound but are still frustrated because they wanted to lose five pounds. I always say to take it one pound at a time. The numbers go 1-2-3-4-5-6, not 2-4-6-8 or 5-10-20. One pound is a lot, and you have to remember CPP. You have to have patience.

QQ involves making a little pattern for yourself. Make it quality of food or quantity of exercise. You need to know what you are eating. Ninety percent of the people don't know how much they eat regarding the total fat, the sugar, the sodium. I always say that people who are in shape are the people who read labels. I've been reading labels for three or four years, and that's helped me a lot. When you put gas in your tank, you have a choice: buy the cheapest one or buy the expensive one. One or the other is going to be better for your car. Some cars have to have regular gas, and some cars, like my car, have to have premium. People might tell me that three blocks away, the gas is a few cents less, but they're not looking at it in terms of quality. Say it's three cents less, and you have a 15-gallon tank. That's what, a 45 cent savings? You need 45 cents? I say not to look at the pennies and focus on the quality of your moments more.

To have success losing weight, you have to have quality of both exercise and food. Eat well, exercise well, and you're going to have success. In my system, you learn this in your first year. It's impossible to learn this in the first two or three months. Losing weight is not easy, but it's not impossible. Weigh the quality against quantity of food, and quality and quantity of exercise. If you don't have one of the two, or you have the other one, you're going to make a mistake.

Who said that all overweight people are unhealthy? Who sets the standard for what is healthy for people? Healthy people eat. People who don't have a disease eat, but people didn't see me as being healthy when I was 500 pounds. I see plenty of skinny people in the YMCA weighing 120 pounds, and they have bad cholesterol and high blood pressure. So, what's healthy and unhealthy for professional people? What is healthy food? What's unhealthy food? That's another thing. Is unhealthy food the food that makes me gain weight? Unhealthy food is still edible; it won't kill you. Just take the QQ into account.

The typical thing I see that people do is to try to eat healthy and not do enough exercise. When I say *enough exercise,* I don't want to go against the nutritionists and personal trainers who tell you to exercise three days a week for forty-five minutes, but in my experience, that's not enough. How in the world could I have lost 300 pounds working out just three days a week for forty-five minutes? That wasn't enough for me. It depends; every single person is different. A person who needs to lose 10 pounds doesn't need the same exercise as the person who needs to lose 100 pounds. I tell people that the exercise depends on how much you've been eating. The point is to burn everything you eat. My slogan is, "I don't care what you eat. Tell me how much exercise you do."

You cannot tell me that you do not have time to exercise. That's called priorities. You need to have priorities and stick to them. As soon as you make a decision to try and lose weight, you have to be professional about it. Make a schedule for exercise. You have to work to make habits, so set yourself up for ninety days, six months, even one year. Unless you do it for six months, it's not a habit. If you miss one day, you have to go back again to day one.

So, we've talked about balancing eating and exercising, and your total calorie package. So, to do it the right way, how much exercise do you need? To lose a pound, maybe half an hour a day is enough. But to lose 10, 20, even 100 pounds, it can't be one hour a day. It has to be more, if it's walking or swimming (perhaps a strenuous exercise such as running would require less time, although it would put more stress on your joints). For most people who have to lose between 20 and 50 pounds, the minimum has to be 2 hours of walking. I don't say to kill your body doing a lot of hard work in the gym that makes 2 hours seems like 4. Just be consistent. If you swim or walk one hour a day in the first month, you'll see results. The first year, you'll see more results. By 8 years, I saw 300 pounds go away. I still don't do anything differently. I keep track of my calories and exercise; that's it.

If you physically get tired, ask yourself if you are trying to do too much exercise. When I have people who try to lose 10 or 15 pounds in a month, of course their bodies get physically tired. But if you're talking about the other kind of tired, the kind when you're tired of doing the same thing, know that you have to find motivation every day. Remember I told you about my scale? I have motivation, every day. Every single day of your life is going to be different. I don't see anyone in America who can say that yesterday was exactly the same day as today. It might look the same, but it's never exactly the same. My motivation, which helps me avoid boredom, is the scale. It's a reminder of my why. Unless you tell me that you get bored sleeping, or you get bored eating, or you get bored going to the bathroom, you can't let yourself get bored with exercise. If you get bored of that, then you're in trouble, but you cannot get bored or tired of something that you decide is crucial to being alive.

Remember the last finger. You use four fingers together: eating, going to the bathroom, sleeping, and exercise. They go together, and you cannot get tired of that. You get tired if you don't see results. When you don't see results, you get frustrated, but if you get frustrated, it's because you don't have patience or you haven't been completely consistent. In all the scenarios that people bring to me, I can tell them why they aren't losing weight. I see you every day in the gym, and you're not losing weight. It's one simple reason: you don't follow how much you're eating in relation to how much you're burning. I live in Tampa, so it's impossible, with a half-tank of gas in my car, to go to Miami. I have to put in more gas, maybe even twice. You need to know how much you have to burn to lose weight.

Chapter 7

Technology: It's there for you to use

Some professionals tell you not to, but I say to use the technology available to help you count your calories, at least for the first year or two years until you feel you're an expert. You're an expert when you have success. My first recommended step is that you should know what you're eating within the first 6 months of starting your program. My favorite app is My Fitness Pal, which helps you keep track of all the food that you eat during the day as well as all the exercise that you do. You eat whatever—pancakes, pizza, healthy food, whatever it is—and you put in there. At the end of the day, it tells you if you pass your package or if you're under your package. If you're trying to lose, you want to be under your package. The next day it will tell you that you did a good job yesterday, and you'll have 300 or 400 calories in your bank. If you imitate that for two to five days in a row, you're going to lose one or two pounds. I recommend this because it works 100 percent. When it doesn't work, it's because you haven't used it properly.

In this sense, cars are almost perfect. Cars know if your temperature gets hot, or if your gas is going down. Cars know the speed. Cars even have a "check engine" light to warn when something is wrong. What do human beings have? Nothing. Just feelings. *I feel full. I feel hungry. I feel tired.* But we don't have a gauge to know it; we don't have a meter. That's why you can eat anything, but you need to know how much you're eating. Healthy or unhealthy, you still need to know how much. And then, you have to know how much exercise you must do. The most common mistake that people make as soon as they start the system is that they don't track calories in versus calories out.

"Danny," they say, "I do exactly what you tell me, but I don't see results."

"Let's see, what are you eating?" I ask.

"Well, I ate this and that."

"Let me see your journey."

"Oh, I didn't follow that."

"Well," I tell them, "that's why."

People might say it's too much to count all the calories, but it doesn't seem like too much when you're going to eat them. As soon as you eat, it takes you ten seconds to put it in My Fitness Pal, and then you know how much you're going to burn. I might see you in the YMCA going for forty-five minutes on the trail, but how do you know if that's enough to burn what you're eating? You need to know, and that app, My Fitness Pal, is amazing. You're going to be addicted to it.

If you go to a restaurant, put in the name of the restaurant, and they have all the menu items, all you have to do is click what you're eating. If, at the end of the day, you go negative, you know that the next day you have to do something. I recommend this app for at least the first year so you know what you are eating. As soon as you pass the first year, you'll be eating almost the same thing almost every day. People don't change their food 365 days a year. Rather, people are generally pretty consistent in what they eat from day to day, and the computer keeps whatever you put in on a daily basis. So you just put in whatever you ate for breakfast, for snacks, for lunch, for dinner, and then track your amount of exercise. In my case, I did lots of swimming, and then I started walking. All I have to do is click those options, and that's it.

I've had success because I would follow what I was doing. When you don't have success in my system of losing weight, it's because you don't follow one of the two recommendations I have: exercising regularly, and making sure you don't surpass your "package" of calories and gain weight. You don't know how much you're eating because you don't write it out, and you need to know. It's like your car. People watch as the gas pump indicates the number of gallons to know how much is going into their cars; or, they pump until the car is full, then leave. You need to know how much you're putting in your system. Never forget that there's nothing you can eat that can make you die. But if you leave it in your system, that's how you'll gain.

So, we're starting to build our case for successful weight loss. First, you need to know your why: why do you want to lose weight? Then, once you know the why, you need to remember CPP. Consistency has to be part of your first day, and you'll need commitment to change something in your life if you want to have success. I don't care why you do, but if you don't change—and that word for me is very strong—you're not going to see results. Part of the reason people who don't have success in losing weight is because of lack of motivation and a lack of information. Perhaps they saw something on TV, and now they want to start losing weight without truly knowing why or how. It took me almost 4 months to prepare myself for my change. It clicked for me when God told me we would do it together, but even before that, He saw me checking on the Internet about people in this country who are overweight. I was checking why people fail, and why they change so much from one thing to another in the world of diet and exercise. I think most people are not prepared to do it, so they come to the professional people, but that's a big business. At the end of the day, they want your money.

Don't do that anymore. You don't have success because you lack a lot of the stuff that you need to do this, so let's start from scratch. From today on, forget everything you did in your past. I don't care what you did in your past. The past is your past. Let's start fresh today. Clear your brain and forget what you did. Forget the mistakes that you made, forget your previous failures. A lot of people lose weight and then gain it back. All this stuff, forget it. Let's start from scratch. Why do you want to change your life by losing weight? I cannot tell you any more if you don't know the why. If you tell me the why, then we can start doing the right stuff. What you did in your past didn't work, and that's why you're here.

My own success in losing weight was like preparing for my dream. It's like I was going to college, and in the history of college, no one graduates in one day, or one week, or two weeks. This is forever. That's why I tell people to forget the goals, because this is going to be forever.

Chapter 8

What motivates you?

Your motivation comes from the power of your brain. Even if you are a negative person, I can convert you to the power of positive thinking for at least one hour because I'm a good motivator. Every single person has motivation, and there are three kinds of motivations in life. For example, when you light a match, the little fire burns for about five to ten seconds. It was fire, but it only burned for five to ten seconds. Like the match, some people motivate for one day, one week, or for one month. Others want the motivation of a candle. Instead of five seconds, candles burn for two or three hours. Those hours represent maybe the two or three months when people start to change, but they start the first month strong, then are less strong in subsequent months before dropping the change they so desired in the early stages.

I'd like to motivate people as if they are torches, rather than candles or matches. I'd like to see them stick with what they are doing for longer, and with more intensity and seriousness.

Every Olympics begins with lighting a torch, and that torch represents how your motivation is forever. Your motivation has to be like a torch, with a strong flame that burns for a long time. It burns despite the enemy. The enemy is the one who says you can't lose weight and will be fat forever. The torch is tall, always, and is very high so no one can reach it.

I've always been a motivator, since I was a little kid. I don't want you to be a match. I don't want you to be a candle. I want you to be a torch.

Most people only feel motivated to make a change for a short period of time. For example, people feel motivated to impress when they start a new job. Check in with these people after the first week, the first month, or the year. After these periods of time have passed, and the initial "glow" of the new job or the new mission has passed, does the motivation remain the same? Probably not. That's human nature.

Many people say, "Danny, you're always happy. How can you do that?"

I see life differently than most, but I'm not a robot. I'm a human being, too, so if I can do it with all the mistakes that I've made in my life, then so can someone else. I don't make the same mistake twice. I see life as good, and I find motivation in it everywhere. You have to have motivation in life, and it can come from your kids, your husband, or your wife. If you don't have it, where are you going? That's part of the reason why people fail. It's a lack of motivation.

When your motivation starts to fade, you need more gas to keep up the flame. You have to connect to the people who motivate you. Don't connect your flame to the people who don't motivate you. Avoid negative people who might try to tell you that you should try this diet or try that gimmick. I say to try to keep at it alone. No one is going to walk for you, no one is going to swim for you, no one is going to exercise for you, and no one is going to eat for you. You do it yourself, and you must think of yourself when you try to keep that motivation strong. It's your change. You have to change yourself every day. Check on the little details regarding what day you have today, what you're going to do today. Plan your day; I love to plan days. I know what I'm going to do tomorrow, and I know what I'm going to do the next day. Always get involved with exercise. Be desperate about it. Take the feeling of being desperate to go to your job or desperate to go to sleep, and try to get involved on that level with your exercise.

Always concentrate on your future, and don't concentrate on your past. People concentrate on the bad days. People concentrate on the fact that maybe two years ago, they tried to lose weight with pills or whatever. Don't focus on that. Motivate yourself. Think of how you're going to look. Get involved with a person who motivates you. Put in a video that motivates you. Always get motivated, and that motivation will change your life. If you change your life, you will see results. If you see results in your favor, you're going to be happy, and you're going to communicate that motivation to other people. I inject motivation into every day. Maybe someone is a match, maybe a candle, but most of my people are a torch. They are very strong.

Motivation is like the fuel of your car. You can have the best car on the planet, but if the car does not have gas it is never going to move. How much gas will you put in your brain? How much gas will you put in your heart? The more motivation you put in your heart, the brighter your torch will burn, and the more results you'll see. In front of me, I already see those who have a big, bright flame activating their torch. Do you know what these people are doing right? Motivating other people as well.

Like motivation, conviction is very important. If you don't believe yourself, you're going to fail. If you don't believe why you do what you do, you're going to fail. You're going to make mistakes in life because no one is perfect. The only perfect thing in this world is numbers. Numbers don't lie. If you aren't a number, and you're a human being, you're going to make a mistake. But, try to learn from that mistake. Conviction is something that you have to have. You must believe in whatever you're doing, and you have to have that conviction from day one. You're overweight now because of something that you've done for a long time, but you've made a decision to lose weight. Conviction has to be always daily, always strong. That's part of my CPP. You must have consistency in conviction, persistence in conviction, and patience.

I guarantee you that people find success in life. Sometimes you don't see it, but just having a job is a success. Having a baby is a success. Having a wife is a success. Having a car, having your house, having yourself, that's success too. People don't pay attention to the little details, which for me are the biggest details. To me, conviction to me is such a big deal. I have so much conviction in whatever I do, and I've done so much stuff in my life.

My doctor told me, "You've got muscular dystrophy; you're going to die in five years."

My conviction said, "No. I'm going to live for my kids. I'm going to live for my life."

That was almost 17 years ago. I have so much conviction that I surpassed that 5 years three times over. Conviction is when nothing negative can control your brain. Nothing. Conviction is everything. If you've got conviction, you're going to have success. It's impossible to fail with conviction.

Negative people are always going to try to be in your way. This is true for business and work as well as your personal transformation or relationships. This life has a lot of negative people, and it could be for any reason that they are negative. But, to convert negative people to positive people, it must be a habit. It's difficult, but it's not impossible. I'm an extremely positive person. I like to tell people that problems don't exist. Think of any problem that you have right now. It could be a tiny problem, it could be a big problem, or it could be a huge problem. I'm going to give you one minute to think of any problem that you have right now. For me, the definition of a problem is something that you feel you cannot resolve. Now I'm going to give you four words, Daniel's magic words: money, time, health, and love. Is your problem one that can be resolved by one of these four words?

Almost 100 percent of people say, "Yes, I can resolve it."

"Then it's not a problem," I reply, "it's a situation."

There are problems, and problems are negative for you to have all the time. You have to see your problems as a result of positive stuff. Problems don't exist because if you can resolve them, it's not a problem. The only problem that truly exists is when you die. Then, there are no problems related to money, no problems related to time, and no problem related to love. There will be no more problems related to health. Know that you can resolve it, and bingo! That's it.

Take the negative people out of your system. Sometimes, they'll be people who are close to you. It could be friends or a part of your family. It could be your husband, your wife, or your kids saying, "Mommy, I like you fat." No, no, no. We have to convert the negative stuff to positive stuff. It's a process, and it's not easy, but remember my definition of habits—you have to have it for over a year. You have to be consistent, persistent, and patient. You're going to have negative people all your life. Usually, these people are either jealous of something you have or something you are. You have to avoid all the negative people because you can convert to a negative mindset yourself when you learn it from someone else. I haven't found any babies so far who are negative—until they're one, two, or three years old and start getting involved with society. That's why the kids start getting stronger, better, or they start to get worse. But, from zero to one or two years old, they're angels. Every day, in all the places you go, you're going to see negative people and positive people. Try to involve yourself with positive people because that's going to help you a lot with your success.

CPP is very important. If you have only two out of three words, though, you're going to fail. I try to be honest with people. Like I said, I don't want to teach; I want to share what I did. I did my CPP since day one, and I still have motivation. I've got plenty of support now. I've got three grandkids, and when I started this journey, I had one. He's watching me now and giving me thumbs up because I'm doing well. That's motivation. I've got two more grandkids now, and it's a blessed life that I have. It's very blessed, and I try to share my blessings. I have a commitment to God to help all the people that He put in front of me. We work together, God and I. I cross people sometimes walking by myself on a trail, and I think, *That's God. He put that lady here for me to help.* That's a miracle.

Every single day of my life, I talk about my story. In my job, I'm a driver, and I have to talk to people on their way to the airport. It's amazing how much lack of motivation I see in this country. If I have to say why that is, I think it's because of society. I always tell people that this life is very; it's us, people, that make life complicated. Each and every one of us has an equal chance to attain success. We all have 7 days a week, 365 days a year, and 24 hours in a day. That's for everybody.

When people say they don't have time to lose weight, I say, "Hold it, hold it, hold it. Stop. I believe you've got twenty-four hours like I do; like Obama, Bill Gates, and your daughter do. Everybody has twenty-four hours." I don't believe that anyone is busy for twenty-four hours every day.

Chapter 9

My involvement with the YMCA

I'm very involved with our local YMCA. It started about seven years ago when I began losing weight, which was in December of 2006. My swimming pool, the first place I started exercising, gets a little cold in the winter, so I was looking for a gym with a heated pool. I found a YMCA close to my home, and they offered to let me swim for the whole winter. I didn't know about the YMCA in the United States before, though I knew about the YMCA in Puerto Rico. You just enroll, and then you exercise. It's a whole gym, the YMCA.

I meet a lot of people there. I joined the YMCA after I lost my first 100 pounds, which I lost in my swimming pool. At almost 400 pounds, I was one of the biggest people in the YMCA. At the beginning, I was too shy. I always tried to help people, but I tried to get more involved in my journey first and then try to help people. I never forget that God is my helper. He always puts people in to help, but at the beginning, it was tough. How could a 400-pound guy help someone when they weigh less than he does? It took me a while, like the first two or three years, to start meeting people in the YMCA. I was one of the shy people. I would do my couple of hours of exercise and go back home. But as soon as I got to 300 pounds, that's when I started getting friends daily. It's impossible to imagine how many people I've met in the YMCA—new people, old people, people of all ages, all sorts of personalities. That's my major. I meet people every day and in every place I go, from the track and the trails to my job.

Everything I've done so far is local, but I hope to help a much larger number of people. I've been on Fox 13 in Florida, and when I go out, people recognize me as the guy who lost almost 300 pounds. I think, *Oh wow, I'm getting famous.* But I want to touch people. I want to tell people how I did it. If I did it with my muscular dystrophy, then anyone can do it. As soon as I meet people, I always try to ask them what they are doing. Almost every single person is trying to do the same thing: they're trying to exercise and to live a more healthy lifestyle. I try to go deeper into their personality. I try to dig up inside to find out what problem they have that has made them gain weight.

I try to support people by staying with them in the gym, the trail, the track, or even in my van. I've done seminars in my van. As soon as I get around twenty to thirty minutes to talk to someone, I guarantee I can change their lives. It's daily for me; I never know when people are going to need me. God is my salesman, and He puts people there for me to help at any time or any place, so I have to be ready. This morning, I met three people, just by coincidence. The were sitting near me and said, "Whoa, you've got a great body." I told them, "Well, you didn't see me eight years ago when I was 500 pounds." That's a good conversation-starter.

Once I have the opportunity to help someone, I do my speech for them. I just talk about what I did. At the beginning, I take five minutes or so to see what they are doing and then try to help them. I tell them what I did, but I never try to change anything about what they're doing if they're involved privately with a personal trainer or nutrition people. If I see a result, I tell people to keep doing what they're doing. My main words are, "You're doing great, keep doing whatever you're doing. Don't change." But if I see people who say, "Danny, I need help because I don't see any results," that's when I get involved with my system.

It's nothing new; all I can share with people is what I did. People want to lose weight in the easiest way, but the easiest way is not always the way that will last you past a year or two years. Losing weight for me is very easy; that's why I try to get people involved. I don't want them to see weight loss as something impossible. I look at it like this: Say I'm the owner of a company, and I'm going to pay you one penny every day to do the worst job you can think of. You start with one penny, but every day, I'm going to multiply that penny by two. Today you make one penny, tomorrow you make two pennies, and the next day you're going to make four pennies, and so on. By the end of the first week, you're going to make one dollar ($1.27, to be exact), and you're going to work for me for just thirty days in the worst job you can of. Most people say, "Of course I'm not going to do that," because people make decisions so quickly. But are you sure you won't do this job that starts at one penny a day and multiplies by two for just thirty days? Ninety-nine percent of the people say no, but the fact is, they just lost $2.8 million in that one month. If you do the math up to thirty days, that one-penny salary doubles itself to be in the millions. I tell folks they shouldn't have made their decision so fast.

Another trick question I like to ask to prove this point is, "Will you jump from an airplane for 1 million dollars?" Of course, most everybody says no, they won't, because they're going to die. But, I didn't tell them yet that the airplane is on the ground, just five feet up. The point is that people need to know what they are going to do. When you say, "I'm going to lose weight," you have to discover your path like I did. I spent three months checking stats, checking knowledge. Ask yourself, *How am I going to change? Am I going to do it fast? Am I going to do it slow?* It's the race of the turtle versus the rabbit. I decided to be the turtle because I didn't want my skin sagging. I discovered that if you do it too quickly, your skin falls. You see my skin now, and you don't see a person who lost 300 pounds.

You don't have to be smart to make a decision. People make decisions in every single second of their lives. Every single day, you make decisions. Sometimes they are quick decisions, sometimes bad decisions, sometimes good decisions, but people have to make decisions. Making the decision to lose weight is something that you cannot do in one day. You have to think about it. I think those who make decisions too quickly are the ones that fail. You have to check it out first. Remember the penny job. Don't tell me you don't want a terrible job that only lasts 30 days if it pays millions of dollars. That's why I tell people to ask questions.

When you get stuck, then you have to change your habits. If you usually do something first, do it last, and your metabolism will think you're doing something different. I change my habits every 3 months. I change my exercise, I change my wake-up call, everything. That's why I've had success for 8 years—I make changes when I get stuck. You have to move. If you move, you'll have success. Learn and move. If you keep learning and keep moving, you're going to have success. That's why God gave you two ears and one mouth: we are supposed to listen. Listen and learn, and you're going to see results. Sometimes they'll be bad results, sometimes they'll be good results, but they will be results from the decisions you make. You're going to see results tomorrow from the decisions you make now. Your life is all about decisions; everything in your life is about decisions. You made a decision in your past, and you're now overweight because you made that decision. No one was born 200 pounds overweight. If you are overweight, it was because of your decisions. You have to make your decisions the smart way. Don't make the penny decision quickly and say, "Nope, I don't want to do that job," because you just lost out on $10 million. People make decisions too quickly. Make a good decision, I guarantee you a good result.

Once you are able to change your habits and lose weight, get involved with your story because you are going to change a lot of people around you. You are going to be a great example. Many people get frustrated or unmotivated because they revert to the same patterns that they have been engaging in for their entire adult lives. The more years you have, the more patterns and habits you have. These habits are the most important things to change. You have to say, *Well, I sleep every day, I eat every day, and I go to the bathroom each day. No one has to tell me I have to go to the bathroom. I can exercise every day.* You might say to yourself, *I was too tired to exercise yesterday. I was so busy with my job.* What, do you work twenty-four hours? It doesn't work like that. That's not conviction.

You can take the pills, you can do all the dieting, but if you don't move yourself, what's going to happen? Babies eat healthy and gain because they don't move. Every day you have to change your habits to stay motivated. At night before you go to sleep, you say to yourself, *Tomorrow, I'm going to do more. I did 20 laps in my swimming pool; I'm going to do 25. I walked 5 miles—let's see if I can walk 6.* Try to improve yourself using your mind, sleep on it, and the next day you have to be motivated. As soon as you go back again to your routine, to your habit, to your family, to your eating, that plane is going down and down and down. You have to dream a lot, and you have to think a lot about what is going to happen to you. When I passed 400-something pounds, I saw myself like I am now: helping the maximum amount of people I can and changing the lives of many. It's frustrating to see people going down after one day or week of motivation.

It's amazing when I walk or swim with people who I talked to one year ago, and their flame is still burning. My biggest frustration is people who don't have a reason why. I have yet to meet a person that I couldn't motivate by speaking to them for a half an hour. I motivate every single person who speaks to me personally. But what happens after that? I think the main reason people fail is because they go back to their routine. When you go back to the routine, that's when your decisions start getting weaker and weaker. I ask people, *what's the difference between yesterday and today? Yesterday I saw you super-motivated. I don't see you for two days, and in two days it's gone?*

I just try to motivate that person with whatever they are doing. If I know the person is making mistakes—and about 90 percent of the people who try to lose weight make mistakes—that's when I get involved and try to share my story. I never teach people, I just share my story. I just tell them what worked for me because I've had a lot of success losing weight. I never try to change the person or whatever they are doing because at least they're doing something. I tell them they're doing great, because at least they're doing something. Whenever a person changes their habits, they're going to see results. But, if they are doing something that I know they aren't going to have success with, I tell them straight. I get involved and tell them with what I did in my life.

Chapter 10

Metabolism, or "yo-yos"

Metabolism hates it when you start doing something right and then you stop. I call it yo-yos, the people here in America who want to lose weight. I lose 10 pounds, then gain 15. I lose 100 pounds, but then I gain back 80. That yo-yo is a simple equation—you start losing weight, you stop, and then you get it back. That little curve is because you betrayed your metabolism, and you betrayed your metabolism because you lost focus on what you're doing. If you're doing something right, keep it up! Why do you have to stop? Keep it up. Find a why, and keep it up forever. It can't be one day or one year or twenty years. It has to be forever.

Then go back to your roots. In business, when your company is successful and doing great, and then something drops, you check why you dropped. If you don't find a reason why you want to do this, it's hard to do, so wait until you find a why. Why do you want to get married? You have to have a reason, right? People have a lot of reasons for getting married, but if it's a weak reason, that's the kind of thing that causes divorce. People forget what they're doing. That's why knowing why you're doing this is important at the beginning. As soon as you start getting results, people love you so much, and they want to see your results, so the why is on another level. But if you don't find the why in the beginning, I'm sorry, but it's going to be tough.

Finding support is key in losing weight, especially when the support comes from your family. If you have support, I guarantee you will have success. Even if, say, you're a single person and no one can support you, you still don't live on this planet alone. If you work, you have co-workers; if you have family outside of your home, that counts as your support. The best support you can have is your mind. Your brain and your mind are something that must work together. People think that the brain and the mind are joined together, but in fact they don't always cooperate with each other. Think of the mind as being the one that maybe thinks you can't do something, the emotional one, but the brain tells you *you can do this.*

Dreams come as soon as they pass from your brain to your heart. Dreams come true as soon as you want them to come true. If you leave your dream in your head, I guarantee it's going to stay in your head. Most people on this planet are unable to make their dreams come true because they leave them in their head; they don't work hard enough to bring the dream to their hearts and into the world. The negative stuff will come, but when faced with people who don't give you support, you have to say to yourself, *Keep going, keep straight.* Look toward the end of the tunnel; don't mix in the middle.

Success doesn't come perfectly; you have failures. You fail at success. A lot of companies fail a number of times. JC Penney went out of business seven times. Amway Corporation went bankrupt roughly four times, and now they have success. Even McDonald's has had its ups and downs. Big companies have success even though they fail sometimes, and you will too. You have to focus on your goals, and your support always has to come from you first. Your family will support you as well because when you do something for your betterment, for your health, you do it for them too. So if you have kids, it's for your kids. But you have to get involved with them—don't lose weight by yourself. Even if your husband is healthy, and your kids are healthy, and you're the only one overweight, get involved with them. "Hey, honey, help me. Don't let me sabotage myself. I need to walk; please come with me." Get involved in your journey, because you never know when you're going to stop.

Chapter 11

Goals

I may be a crazy person, but I don't trust in goals, aside from staying focused on what you want. Why is that? Because a goal is something that when you hit it or you reach it, then you stop, but the goal here has to be forever. Remember the CPP acronym from earlier, particularly the "persistence" part.

I talk mostly to obese people, people who are at least 75, maybe 100 pounds over their limit.

When people who fall into this group tell me they have to lose some large amount of weight (say, 20 pounds), I smile. Always.

"What? Are you crazy?" I say. "Lose five pounds first. Twenty is too much. Start with five." Then I explain what I did.

When I was 500 pounds, my goal was 480, then 460. In my case, I had to lose more than maybe the average person in America needs to. For me, it was every 10 or every 20 pounds, but the maximum was 20, no more than 20. For people who have to lose 20, 30, or 50 pounds, don't say 50. The goal is 5 pounds.

I have success with people who say, "I remember I told you I had to lose 80 pounds, and I thought I'd never lose 80. But you told me to do it in smaller portions like 5 pounds, and I've already come so far."

Goals are something I don't like to talk about because when you don't reach a goal, what happens? You feel frustrated. That's why on January 1, a lot of people set goals, and then in February or March, they're frustrated because they've failed at that goal. Don't set goals. Get the support of your family, and know that this is forever. I don't like to make goals. Goals are for candidates or athletes, people who aim to win a race, the World Series, or a championship game. Those are goals. But on a personal level, I don't like to set goals because nine out of ten people are going to fail, and that failure can sabotage their entire dream.

Something I also discovered is that we don't know when we're going to die. It could be tomorrow, the coming Wednesday, next month; 2020 is coming, 2050 is coming, and we don't know if we're going to be there or not, so don't concentrate on the finish line. The finish line is the day you die, and you don't know when that day might be. I prefer people to say, "Support me all you can because I don't have any goals."

In my case, I never thought that I would make it to 185 pounds. Never. Never in ten lives. I remember I woke up from my dream when I passed 400. When I saw 390-something, I thought, *Oh, my gosh*. I never put that goal on myself. I was just engaging in the same weight-loss behaviors that I was without making goals. I was swimming more, maybe walking more, and I found myself continuing to lose weight. I remember being at 300 pounds. When I got stuck at 300, I really started moving. *Let me walk*, I thought, *just walk and swim*.

I remember people telling me, "Danny, 250 is enough. You look great."

"No," I'd tell them, "let me enjoy my healthy way."

Nutritional experts say for a six-foot-tall person, you should be 170 to 190 pounds, and that's an average. I wanted to feel it. I remember it took me almost a year to go from 220 to 210 pounds, but when I saw the 210, I thought maybe I could be 200. Today, when people ask me if I'm going to stop, I say, "No. I don't know if I'm going to die today, but if not, I'm going to continue." So, it is possible for goals and support to almost get together. Support me with no goals.

"Danny, where is all your skin after your 300-pound loss?" That's the first reaction that almost everyone has when they see me.

When I was on Fox 13 News, I told Doctor Joe, "I believe the skin is the dumbest part of your body. The skin doesn't know what you do, so you can fool it. My weight loss was the race of the rabbit and turtle, and we all know who won that race? It was, of course, the turtle. I decided I was going to start losing weight very slowly, so when I started losing weight in the water, my skin started shrinking at my speed. It took almost 7 years."

I've broken some pretty amazing and impressive records. As I look back on the journey of my life so far, I realize that God prepared me since day one to have success in life. I look back 45 years and think, *wow, that's why I've had success in life. Look at what I did when I was 5 years old.* I started in the private school in my town in Puerto Rico, which my younger brother and my 2 sisters also attended. I went there from kindergarten to eighth grade.

At eighth-grade graduation, the principal announced, "We have an amazing accomplishment here. This little kid has a record that no one in this school is going to break. His name is Daniel Alvarez, and from kindergarten to eighth grade, he never missed one day of school. He was never late, not even for one minute, for school. He was never absent, and he never missed any day of school."

I was freaking out with excitement. Maybe people say that's not impressive, but most little kids get sick or miss an appointment or something, while I never did. I've been honored to have the trophy of perfect attendance from kindergarten to eighth grade, and it didn't stop there. In ninth grade, I started in another private school in Puerto Rico for high school. In the four years between ninth grade and senior year, I never missed one day, and I never was late. That's consistency. When I ran my own company in Puerto Rico, I doubt I missed one day, because I love to be the first one in everything. My family says I'm the super-responsible guy. In anything I do, I have to be the first one. I go to my job now at four or five o'clock in the morning because I have to be the first one.

I'm so responsible that on June 1, 2013, I saw thirteen years working in the hotel without missing one day, without calling off, without making excuses or being late. I've had perfect attendance almost my whole life. I call that consistent. It's an impressive record, and I apply the same level of consistency to my weight loss. In eight years, I haven't missed one day—one single day—of swimming or walking. I don't care if I'm on vacation, I still do it, and I go on vacation with my family and grandkids to Orlando almost every month. Even there, I have to swim or I have to walk.

All these records of consistency are amazing, but that's what people have to do. It's part of your life. Consistency means doing it every single day. You do all kinds of things every single day, but you don't pay attention to them. You don't know what you've been doing every day since you were born, but it's definitely included eating, sleeping, and going to the bathroom. If you can do that, just add one more thing. We're capable of adding something to our lives on a daily basis, but we don't pay attention to that. I always say that exercise has to be there like my sleeping, like my eating, like going to the bathroom. No one tells you to do that.

Your conviction has to be consistent, persistent, and patient from day one. You need to be professional. Losing weight can't be like you're going to the park to play baseball. Losing weight means you have to do it the professional way. The maximum is 300 pounds and the minimum is one pound to be professional. One pound or 300 pounds, you need to know calories in versus burning calories. If you don't know, what's going to happen? You're going to be eating very healthy and then doing a half-hour of exercise, and in 2 months, you're gaining weight. Boom! Fail. That's 9 out of 10 people.

When you start doing it the right way, which is the way that I like to share, try to count for the first two years. Get involved. Be professional. My graduation for people is one year. If you're doing something, just do it for one year and see what happens. When people tell me they've been trying to lose weight for three months, I'll tell them to give me a week to see results. In one week people say, "Wow, that's good," and I'll tell them to multiply that by more. Multiply those results by 1 month, and then by 2 months, and then by 3 months. We don't have a gauge or a meter to tell us how much we're eating, so we have to count. Now, with all the technology that we have, it's easier. Whenever you go to fast food, they have to tell you the nutrition facts. The restaurant has to tell you the nutrition facts. The computer has a nutritional chart, your phone has a nutritional chart, any place you go, any place in the world, has a nutritional chart. As soon as you know how much you're eating, you know to burn it off the next day.

The second most asked question is, "Danny, I'm exercising, but I'm not losing. What happened?"

That's why I tell you to follow whatever you're eating. Do the calorie counting. It's up to you for how long you do this; no one knows your body better than you. No one else knows the type of food that you eat that makes you gain like you do. It might be different for different people. As soon as you know all the tricks in yourself, that's when I tell people they've graduated, and that's in a year. In a year, you know. Change comes with habit. If you don't follow your calorie counting for at least one year, it's going to be tough because you don't have a super-memory to know how much you ate. I don't regularly follow My Fitness Pal because (by my own criteria) I'm an expert. However, for the first 5 or 6 years of my weight loss journey (until I hit 250 pounds), I was using it every day. So, to put that in perspective, I used it during a period of time when I lost 250 pounds. Now, I follow My Fitness Pal more because you can follow the progress of other people. I can chat with them, say, "Hey, great job today." I'll be able to watch them, seeing their eating and exercise habits. I tell people it's a process that lasts forever if it's done the professional way. I prefer that way.

The other question I'm often asked is how I did it, and I tell people I did it all with my mind. Your mind is the one that tells you, "Do it," or "Don't do it," or "How am I going to do it?" If you don't clear your brain first before you make that decision, it's going to be very difficult.

People ask me, "Do you have to do exercise every day? The experts tell me three or four times per week for a half-hour is all I need."

"Sorry," I say, "that's for normal people, not for obese people."

If you eat every day, sleep every day, and go to the bathroom every day, why can't you do exercise every day? I guarantee you no one on this planet doing exercise three times per week for half an hour can lose 300 pounds like I did. It depends on how much you eat that tells you how much exercise you're going to do. People change when they understand my system. It's almost opposite to what the professionals tell you, but it's a more reasonable way than the professional opinion. The professionals always go straight to the best thing, but for that to work, they would've had to tell me about it when I was five years old. Now, I'm fifty years old, I talk to a lot of people who are seniors, or who are 30 and 40 years old. It's tough to change your life when you've had a pattern, a system, for years.

Another question is, "Danny, what do you eat?"

Eating is not my problem. I focus on how I'm going to take the eating out of my system. The only way is to jump in my pool or walk through the trail or going to the Y. I have to be honest: I eat anything I want to. Anything I want to eat, I eat. I don't suffer eating. People who suffer eating are almost everybody who diets, and then the next morning they say, "Oh, last night I wanted to eat a little cake." What's my answer to these people? Eat it! Eat it, and start burning it off today or tomorrow.

I don't want to take food from anyone's system like the nutritionists do. I don't want to do that, because once you make that decision, how long are you really going to keep it? Would you put your son out of your house, or your husband? What if I said you should try and new husband or a new kid? What do you think would happen?

People ask me, "Danny, can I do this diet?" referring to the latest diet craze.

I always say the same thing: "Are you going to do it for the rest of your life? If the answer is no, don't do it."

You can be a master eater as soon as you know how you are going to do it. I know how to do it, but I want people to know how to do it for themselves. I eat anything I want, but the more I eat, the more I have to exercise. The less I eat, the less exercise I have to do. Your intestines are very long, so God gave you enough time to burn what you eat. Don't leave it for more than twenty-four hours, and you won't fall behind. Why suffer while you are eating? One of the most common reasons that people fail is because they desire the goodies they can't have. God told me that we are capable of burning anything. There's no food on the entire planet that we cannot burn.

Chapter 12

Recognizing the journey

I started receiving recognition for my journey around this time last year. I was exercising in the YMCA and started chatting with the person next to me. We were talking about life, and he asked me if I was losing weight at that moment. I told him I'd actually lost a lot of weight. At that time last year, I had lost almost 280 pounds, so I was maybe 220 or 230 pounds, and he got impressed with that. He was almost interviewing me the whole half-hour I was with him. At the end, he told me, "Here is my card," and it turned out he was a reporter for the Huffington Post, and he was on vacation here in Tampa. I'll be honest: I didn't even know what the Huffington Post was at that time. He told me it was the newspaper of the Internet.

"Let me tell you something, Mr. Alvarez," he said. "Your story is so impressive, I would like to get your permission to put it in my column."

"Oh yes, it would be an honor," I replied. "If putting my story in the newspaper is going to help other people, go ahead."

About two months later, they called me to tell me they needed some pictures and that the article would be posted in July. I thought, *wow, that's amazing.* It was almost what I was feeling in my dreams. I was still thinking I was 500 pounds, but then I knew I had really changed.

After that, one of the anchors at Fox 13 loved the article, and they called me at the YMCA because the article said I worked out there. I met the anchor soon after.

"Danny, I've been looking for you," he told me. "When I saw your article, it impressed me so much, the way that you lost weight. Can I have permission from you to do like a short documentary about you?"

"Yes," I said, "it's an honor again."

That was the first time that Fox 13 TV in Tampa went to the YMCA to interview me. It was one of the best feelings when I received the news after they recorded everything that it would be on the air the next Friday. That was August 17, and after August 17, everything started to feel like a dream. I received another call from the anchor from Fox 13.

"Danny, we received over a quarter million hits from Facebook about your article and about your story. Is it possible for you to come on live TV with one of the nutritional doctors on the channel?"

I said yes because if it's regarding helping people, then that's what I'm going to do. Everything starts with one conversation. I have a strong conviction about what I do; everything starts from that. I was on TV two times, and now I'm helping more people. My goal is to help part of the 180 million people that are overweight here with my program.

It feels amazing to receive this kind of attention for what I've done. After being on the air, my motivation is that every time I go to any place, people recognize me as the guy who lost a lot of weight. The more motivated that people see me, the more that becomes my motor to help people. It's a dream come true what happened to me. The Fox 13 spot that they gave me I think was God helping me. He's preparing me for the big impact that we're going to have. I see that coming soon—it's something that I cannot express in words. It's amazing it happened to me so quickly; everything has happened in one year. I've been doing that for seven years, and who can tell me how many years we've got left to help people? It's amazing.

Chapter 13

Healthy food and access

There are two types of food in this world: healthy food and less-healthy food. No food exists that if you eat it, you die (with the exception of food that's contaminated or not cooked properly)—it's not like that. Food is good, and a lot of people don't have food. I think the problem in the US is that healthy food is more expensive than unhealthy food. I believe the government has to be involved. We need the help of the government so that more people can have access to healthy food. It's all about money, and I know this because I'm a business guy. People buy the unhealthy food because it's cheaper, and everything cheaper is less healthy. Why don't we change our policies so that the unhealthy food is more expensive? This would allow healthier food to compete based on price. Why don't we increase the accessibility of healthier food? I guarantee you 100 percent that if we put the super-healthy food on this planet at the prices of the unhealthy food, people will start buying more healthy food.

People buy unhealthy food because that's what they can afford. What a coincidence—the people who are in shape are the people buying the healthy food, and then you go to another grocery store where everybody is overweight, and they're buying unhealthy food. My dream is to see that change a little bit. I've talked to a lot of people who say they cannot buy the healthy food because it's too expensive.

"I have to buy this because it's more reasonable for me. It's unhealthy, but it's all I can afford." I hear this over and over.

I think the government wants people who don't have the access or the tools to buy better food to be overweight. One of the cheapest foods in Puerto Rico for poor people used to be a can of corned beef. When I was growing up in Puerto Rico, a can of corned beef was $.50. That same can of corned beef has gone up to $7.99, and no one can buy that corned beef now. Corned beef is an unhealthy food, and that's what clicked my idea. The government needs to talk to the powers that control the grocery stores and the manufacturers and say, "You know what? Let's start manufacturing more healthy food. Let's put a little twist on the pricing."

Say I go into any fast food joint and see a menu with a hamburger, fries, and a soda for $12.95. Then there's this little salad with grilled chicken for maybe $.99. I want to challenge anyone who goes to fast food restaurants to do that test for one day to see how many people buy the burgers, fries, and sodas for $12.95 or $15.95 versus how many people buy the salad and grilled chicken for $.99. See what happens. The market is against poorer people, and it keeps them unhealthy. People cannot buy the healthy food because it's not affordable, and the people with the resources to buy the healthy food are the healthy people who are in great shape. But, the government won't get involved, because the more people who are heavy, the more diseases they have, the more money the doctors make. That's the sad part of the business, sadder because I think they like it that way.

My wife has worked as a cook at a public school in Tampa for the past fifteen years. She cooks for almost eight hundred kids, and she tells me that each Friday is pizza day at the school. For eight hundred kids, there will be maybe one hundred pizzas and twenty salads with the healthy stuff, and every Friday she tells me, "You know what, honey? Seventeen salads left, and all the pizza is gone." Even kids get started on the unhealthy food because it's more accessible. Why can't we turn the tables and put up the pizza for five dollars and the salads for free just to see what happens for the kids?

In the lobby at my job, we have a check-in just for kids, and they get to write down some facts about themselves like their favorite foods. It's amazing to see the lists—almost every single kid says their favorite foods are pizza, burgers, hot dogs, French fries, macaroni, ice cream, M&Ms, and so on. Listed in front of me are two hundred kids between the ages of six and ten saying they love unhealthy food. Everything starts when you're a kid. So kids love all this stuff—which is cheaper than the healthy stuff—and that's part of why we're going the wrong way. That's why we have to stop the 180 million overweight people in this country another way.

That's the reason I made this book. I'm here to spread the word to say, "Hey, we have to burn calories." If you move, you burn calories. We have time to burn the calories we eat—that's why God gave us twenty feet of intestines. You're capable of burning any food you eat, but it makes a big impact when you eat healthy rather than unhealthy food. I lost 300 pounds not by eating particularly healthy, because to be honest, I'm not one of the ones who is capable of buying the healthy food. I do more exercise so I can eat whatever. I can burn everything with my swimming or my walking, so I don't care what I eat. But I know that in one year, if the government said that all the unhealthy food is going to be more expensive and the healthy food will be cheaper, I know that overweight people will start buying the healthy food. It's simple business logic at work.

I think this country has been overweight for a reason. With all due respect to the professionals, I've come up with my own story of how this country became so overweight. Before all the mega fast food chains started back in the '50s, the status of the United States was decreasing. I imagine the doctors, nutritionists, personal trainers, and psychiatrists meeting one day in an office.

"You know what?" they said. "We're not making business. The war was a couple years ago, the government is going down, and all these countries are better than us. We have to put this country in a situation in which all four of us can make money. If more people get fat in this country, they're going to start getting sick. When they get sick, they come to us."

Say I'm your doctor, and I prescribe you something and tell you to go to the nutritionist. The nutritionist will probably tell you something you don't like because they're going to cut some food out of your system. The food that you buy is cheaper, but they're going to tell you to eat something else to make sure they make their money. In two or three weeks, if you're not losing weight with your diet or something, they're going to tell you to go to the gym where a personal trainer can help you. You start with the personal trainer, but they just tell you some stuff that doesn't really work for you. They've never been and never will be overweight because they're trainers—maybe one trainer out of a million will have been 300 or 400 pounds. They're going to tell you the exercises they know how to do, but the catch is that those exercises are all for healthy people. Then, you begin to get tired, and start to go crazy, and now you're going to the psychiatrist. The psychiatrist is going to tell you more stuff, and all of them are going to make money.

What a coincidence that all these industries evolved at the same time the fast food industry did. That's why something like 120 million more people are overweight in 2013 than in the 1950s. I guarantee you the government could help those who are overweight. Now, pretty much all the fast food chains have healthy options, but the government has to push more incentives for the mega restaurants to put more healthy stuff and less unhealthy stuff on their menus to improve people's access to healthy foods. It's not you, it's not me, it's not normal people who are making the money, but someone out there is making it. I don't want to talk much about the government because I love this country so much. Puerto Rico has been in America for one hundred years, and I love it, but this country is going in the wrong direction.

Never mind the discussion of social security. If you're fat, there's a good chance that when you're 65 years old, you're going to have diabetes, high blood pressure, perhaps a stroke, all because you're overweight. If you make it that long, at the age of 72, you don't have any more social security because your money is gone. From now on, I want to get the government more involved in helping us. There are 180 million overweight people in this country, which makes us the majority of this nation. The majority of this nation is overweight, and the government has to help us confront all this illness.

Chapter 14

Meeting with God

Every day, God and I have meetings. I call them my staff meetings, and it's just Him and me together, every single day, since I made a commitment to Him. All this was His idea. I didn't know. I was gaining weight, and there was no reason for me not to have high blood pressure, high cholesterol, or diabetes, but that was His miracle. He was preparing me for the reason, and every single day I tell Him, "Thank you." He's doing His job, and I'm doing my job. We've been helping people every single day. My relation with Him is the best. He's my partner, He's my life, and without Him, I wouldn't have made it. I promised Him, and He promised me, that this is going to be forever. Maybe it's going to take us 10 years, 20 years, 50 years, 100 years, I don't know, but we're going to get to our people and help them.

My motto is about getting power to explore the world. It seems impossible, but as long as God is with me, I can do anything. I tell people that sometimes He is what you need. Be a part of Him. It's in my system, my partnership with God. If you need help, talk to Him. One way or another, we have hope that we can change people's lives, and you have to appreciate this life so much. God gave you this life, but He didn't tell you when you're going to leave. That's His secret. He knows, but He's not going to tell you because He wants you to live with the maximum amount of happiness in this life. No person that comes to this world leaves this world without making a story of his or her life. Sometimes babies leave, sometimes adults leave, sometimes old people leave, but every single person goes back to Him because they did His job. It's a miracle, what He did for me, and what He's still doing for me.

I was diagnosed with muscular dystrophy in 1993. For almost 10 years, I got worse and worse, until I was in a wheelchair and could only walk using a cane. I was a humble person, and sometimes I didn't go out so people wouldn't see me like that. I was getting a little fatter because all of the medicine and all the stuff that was inside my body. I remember it was Labor Day, and I was watching Jerry Lewis on the muscular dystrophy telethon. I wondered why they hadn't found a cure and thought, *You know what? I'm not a doctor, but I'm going to do it myself, with the help of my doctors.* I appreciate the help my doctors gave me, and I thank God because one of the best doctors for my disease is here in Florida with me.

When I bought this house—and my wife is going to laugh when she reads this—the only thing that God put in my eyes was the swimming pool. We're talking about 15 years ago, when I first came from Puerto Rico and wasn't overweight. I was maybe 200 to 220 pounds. We didn't like our house, but we loved that patio. I love it to this day, and we have such a nice atmosphere out here. It was the swimming pool that God put in my eyes because that was the swimming pool, one day, would save my life.

I told my wife, "Let's buy that house."

"But we don't like it," she said.

"Don't worry," I said, "something is going to happen."

I bought my house in 1998. In 2000, I started with the hotel, and I was normal, but 5 to 6 years later, boom! Five hundred pounds. That swimming pool was what saved my life. As I started to exercise more regularly, my weight was going down drastically. I used to have seven doctors at the University of South Florida, and they were all surprised that I was losing weight. I told them I was going to get stronger. Water is a miracle. Three-quarters of our body is water. And three-quarters of our planet is water. God put a lot of water here for a reason.

Through the years when I was losing more, I was getting a little stronger. I still don't have the same power that I had when I was 17 or 18 years old up to twenty-six years old when they discovered muscular dystrophy in me. My doctors have a scale of one to ten where ten is strong and one is weak, and I spent almost 10 years between two and three. After some months spent exercising, I got up to a five. To everyone's surprise, I'm now between a seven and an eight. I don't have my old level of strength back, but the doctors cannot believe what I did. The water changed my life. I don't know if what I did would help everybody with muscular dystrophy, but for all people, when you have a muscle problem, try the water to see what happens. It helped me. Everybody always told me to go to the Jacuzzi. I know water means something, and for me, I've improved a lot.

I'm a new person. When I go back to Puerto Rico, people cannot believe that the guy who left Puerto Rico twenty years ago in a wheelchair is walking now. I'm getting stronger, and the water did it for me. The walking did it for me too. Eight years ago, I said I would be a new person because I had to get ready to help people. I started this journey with God and my clean brain. I didn't study to be a salesman, I didn't study to be a psychologist, nor did I study to be a doctor, trainer, or a nutritionist. But, I can help people, and I do it for free. In that way, my love for people means more than any kind of money that professional people try to get from you. My doctors still say that I'm a miracle because they've never seen a person weigh 500 pounds without hypertension, high cholesterol, or anything related to diabetes. I was just a big guy; God put me together so I could help as many people as I could.

My doctors say, "Danny, what a change." That's a word that I love: change. Change, love, commitment, conviction, consistency, persistence, those are words I always use in my vocabulary. Try to change yourself. Change your family, but don't do it for them. Do it for you, and I guarantee you they'll be so proud of you that they, too, will get involved. Even if they don't need to lose weight, they're going to get involved. Just change yourself. You cannot change the world, but if you change yourself, maybe you'll change your family. If you change your family, maybe you'll change your neighbors, or your friends. Maybe you'll change your town or your state, and then maybe you'll change the world. I changed myself, and now I'm changing a lot of people.

One time, a lady told me, "Danny, even if I don't lose weight, you changed my life."

Those words were so powerful for me. That's my reason—I want to change the lives of others. I know she's going to do it—she's already lost 60 pounds. It's good to get involved with your family. Tell your family that you're happy and that you're with God. If you're sick, if you have diabetes or high cholesterol, do it for yourself, not because a doctor told you that you have to or you will die. Do it for yourself, and I guarantee that you will see the change of your life and your relatives and your friends and your family and everybody around you.

One day, I asked, "God, what are you doing to me?" because I was tired of being overweight.

He started laughing, and then I started laughing too. "Why are you laughing to me?" I asked.

"You struggle now, but your story is going to change the life of a lot of people," He told me.

I would be happy just to help my daughter, my son, and my grandkids regarding their exercise, but no, that's not my reason for being here. My reason is to help more people. I came to this world to help people, and that's the only purpose of my book. When people read it, maybe they will identify with me, whether they want to lose 5 pounds or 100 pounds. I want them to think, *whoa, this guy lost 300 pounds. I just need to lose 10 or 20. Let's see what he did.* It's simple. Just check the CPP, check the QQ, start moving, start learning, and you can do it.

When I was on TV, I was told, "You're an inspirational story. You inspire people so much," and I was very happy to hear that because that's my goal. People who know me for a while know why I have a master's degree in helping people and a PhD in loving people. It's because I'm always good. Everybody at my job knows that Danny is always good, always happy. I have the same positive attitude. I don't have problems, so if people have problems, they can come to me. If I can resolve it with money, with love, with time, or with health, then it's not a problem. Take that word out of your system. When you think, *I have a problem,* say instead, *I have a situation.* See life differently, and remember to take it one day at a time. Tomorrow is coming, next week is coming, and 2015 is coming—with you or without you. So take it one day at a time, and remember that every single person on this planet came for a reason, and you have to discover that reason with God.

All my family is involved now. I'm very proud of my daughter, who made the decision I made 8 years ago last year, and she's lost 155 pounds with my system. She's 29 years old, didn't really exercise for 28 years, and wasn't eating too healthy. As I've said, if you don't eat healthy and don't exercise, you're going to be overweight. It's something that is part of being a human being. She just made one decision.

"Daddy, I'm ready. Help me," she said.

"Let's start now," I said. "Let's start in the pool."

We started swimming, walking, and drinking more water. She started drinking more water than I'd seen her drink in my entire life. She knows how to drink water. She made a little change, and within a year, she's seen results. She's excited, and my family is excited with her and with me. My wife is getting involved in my scheduling. She receives the calls and reminds me if I have a meeting today. All my grandkids, especially my grandson, are watching me. They love me so much.

My grandson knows he was part of my decision that I made 8 years ago. He's the one that, when he was two, said, "Grandpa, you're so big."

I thought, *you know what? I'm going to lose weight. I have a reason to live. I have a reason to see my grandson grow.* Now, he's going to turn 9 years old. My son is doing a great job as well; he has also changed his life. Every person in my close family sees the success I've had. It's decisions that we have to make every single day of our lives. As soon as we wake up in the morning, we make decisions. *What decision do I have to make for tomorrow? Am I going to lose weight or am I going to stay like I am?* It's your decision.

Make a smart decision, not the decision of the penny. Know why you're going to do it. Remember there are no goals in this system—it's forever, for the rest of your life. You don't know when you're going to die, so don't make goals. That way, you won't get frustrated when you don't achieve a goal. Be patient because it's going to be forever.

Every time my daughter calls me and says, "Daddy, I gained 2 pounds," I say, "Gaining two pounds is awesome, just don't gain 10."

When you're losing weight, gaining 2 to 5 pounds is acceptable to me. This morning at the YMCA, a lady told me she gained 5 pounds, and I told her I thought that was enough. She knows how to dial it back. She graduated from my system; she's already passed one year already. If you don't pass one year, I know have to share more of my story or motivate you more, but I have plenty of gas in my system to share with people. My flame is like a torch, and it could burn for 20 years or more. Make a good decision, and do it for you. Love yourself. Ask God to help you, and He will tell you what to do.

Make a good decision in your life and try it. I'm pretty sure every person who has tried to lose weight has tried 2, 10, 20 different things in their lives. If you're just 5 pounds overweight, maybe you haven't tried much. If you're obese, I'm sure you've tried many things through the years. It might work for one day, but I would like you to try this system that I know works. I've watched so many people change their lives with it. If you like to eat, if you like to exercise, this is for you. If you don't like to eat healthy and you like to exercise, this is also good for you. If you eat healthy and you also exercise, this is also good for you. If sometimes you don't eat healthy or sometimes you don't do exercise, this is also for you. This is for all four kinds of people that we have in this world. With big motivation, people of each of these four types can change their lives, and can also help other people change. Make a decision to move yourself.

When I tell people anything is possible, it depends on if you want it, so you have to make a decision. Make a decision, and have conviction in your life. Imagine how are you going to look 20 pounds lighter or 50 pounds lighter. Love yourself, because no person on this planet besides God loves you more than you do. Love yourself, and do what you have to do. Pray to God and say, *Yeah, we're going to do it.*

Chapter 15

If I had to do it again

If I had to go back again, if someone challenged me to go back to 500 pounds and lose it again, I think I could, but I would have to have a reason first. I don't see where I'm going to get the motivation to go back, though, because in my 8 years, I didn't gain even 5 pounds back. That means that my motivation is like a torch.

I still motivate myself. I open my eyes and say, "Who am I going to help today, God? Yesterday you gave me 10 people. I want more today; I'm ready for more."

I want quality people, I want people who try to get their flame not like the match or the candle; I need torch people. I need people who say, "I can do it. If Daniel did it, I can do it."

Maybe I'm waking up from my dream, but I look back on myself seven years ago, and I'm very honored. My pool is very sentimental to me. That water saw me lose almost 200 pounds. The streets of Tampa saw me lose another 100 pounds, and now, helping people at the YMCA is my goal. Like I said, I don't want to sell anything; I just want to help people. Helping someone else lose weight is who I am; it's why I'm here.

God bless you and don't forget to have success: 'CPP & QQ Consistent Persistent and Patient with the Quality of Food and Quantity of Exercise.

"Dreams come true as soon as you put them into work. Dreams come as soon as they pass from your brain to your heart. Dreams come true as soon as you want them to come true."

"It's impossible to fail with conviction."

Photo Gallery

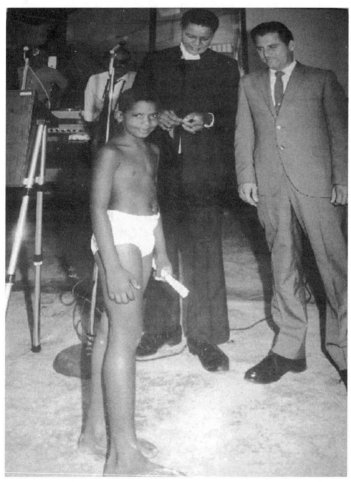

1968: I received my first diploma from swimming

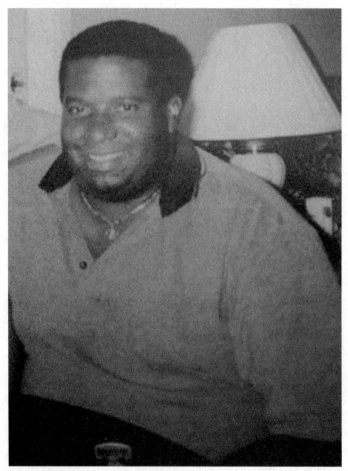

I was gaining weight.

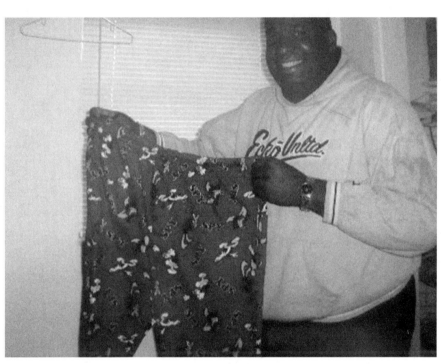

First 100 pounds lost.

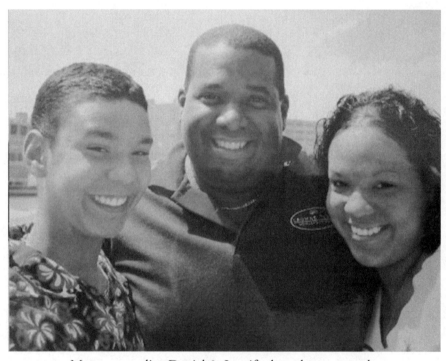

My reason to live Daniel & Jennifer love them so much.

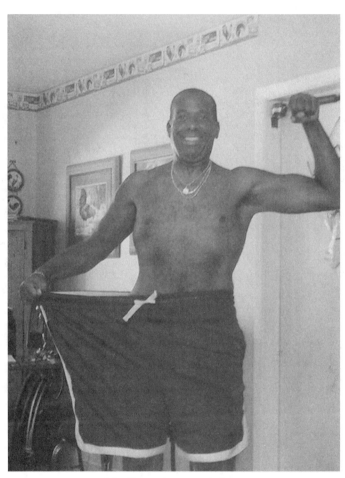

My first 250 pounds lost.

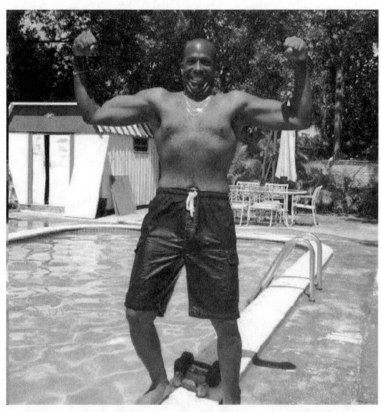

My grandson Keith took that picture to celebrate when I hit 200 pounds.

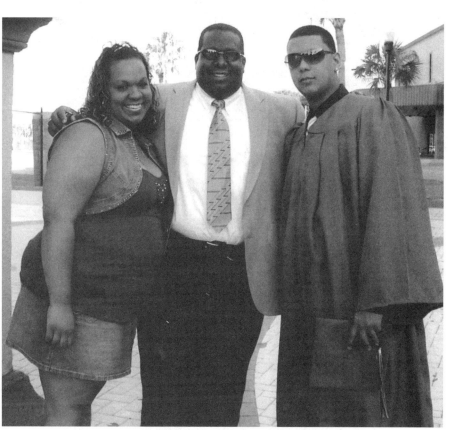

More than 485 pounds. 52-inch waist, 4XXXX shirt.

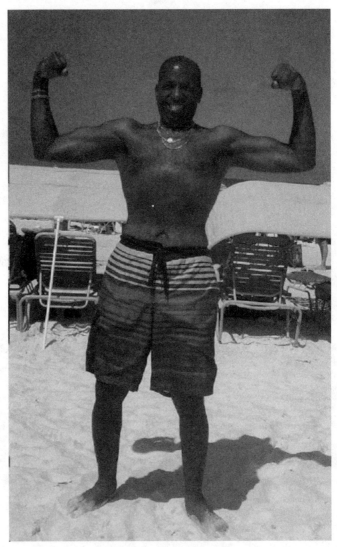

300 pounds lost. 34-inch waist, medium shirt.
Wow! What a change.

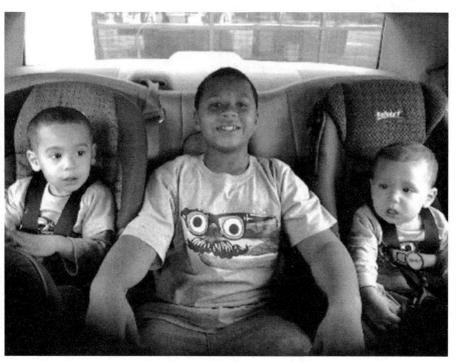

My 3 grandkids Anthony Keith & Kayden
The reasons for my success!

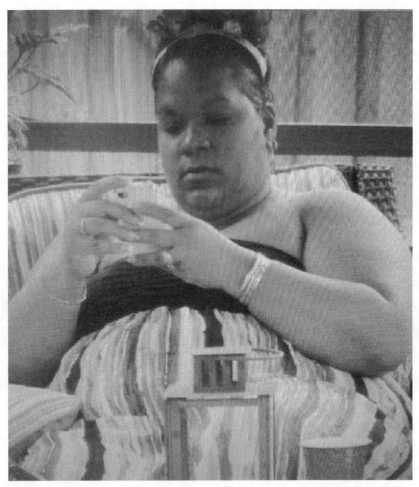

My daughter 400 pounds.

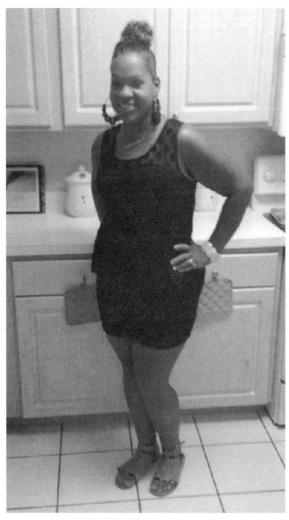

My daughter 175 pounds lost with my system.

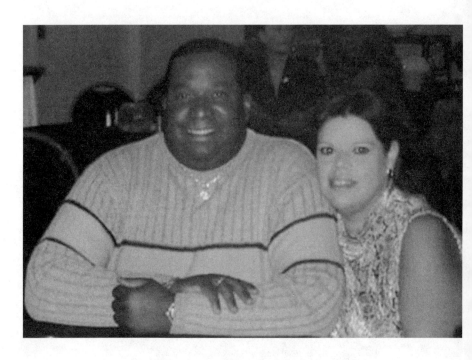

2006

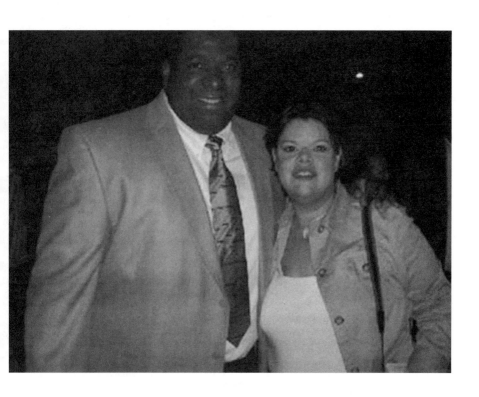

2007

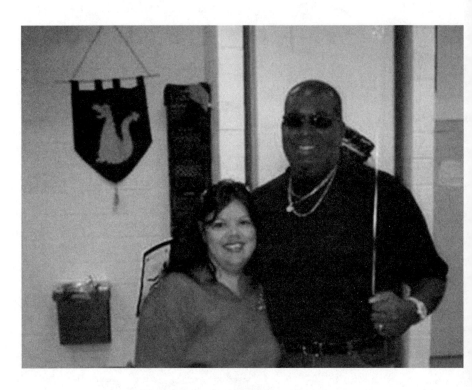

2009

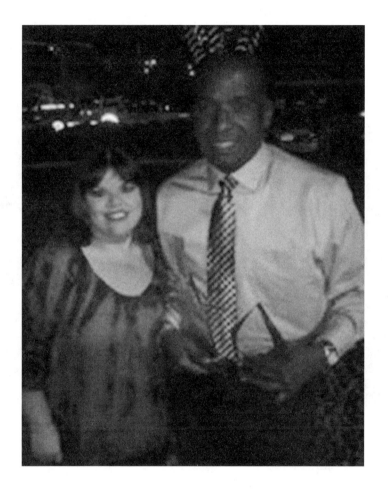

2011

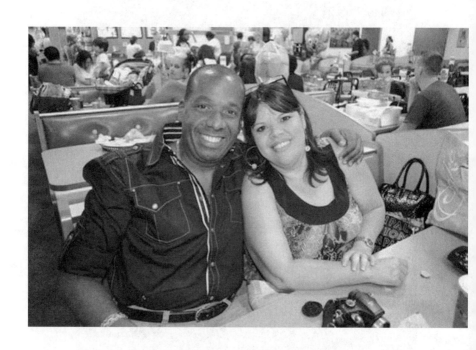

2012

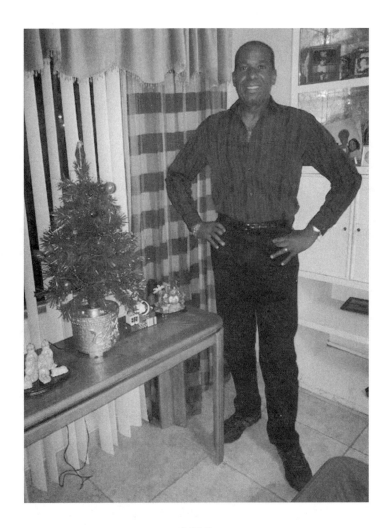

2013

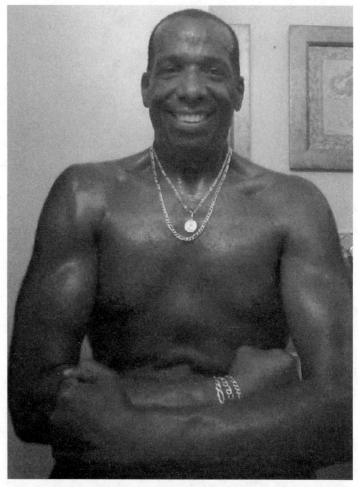

To my readers, if you wish to get in contact with me, send me an email at
DANNY8488@AOL.COM.
I will be glad to share my expertise on how to keep oneself fit.